Rise & Shine

Rise & Shine

EMPOWER YOUR MINDSET, GET FIT, CHANGE YOUR LIFE

TOM TROTTER

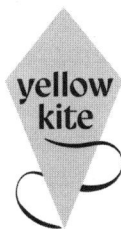

First published in Great Britain in 2025 by Yellow Kite
An imprint of Hodder & Stoughton Limited
An Hachette UK company

The authorised representative in the EEA is Hachette Ireland,
8 Castlecourt Centre, Dublin 15, D15 XTP3, Ireland (email: info@hbgi.ie)

1

This Work was edited by Arielle Steele.
Illustrations © Wioleta Deptula 2025

A CIP catalogue record for this title is available from the British Library

The information in this book is not intended to replace or conflict with the
advice given to you by your doctor or other health professional. All matters
regarding your health should be discussed with your doctor. If you have
any health concerns regarding the fitness plan, we recommend that you
consult with your doctor before you embark on it. The author and publisher
disclaim any liability directly or indirectly from the use of the material in
this book by any person.

Trade Paperback ISBN 9781399753135
ebook ISBN 9781399753142

Typeset in Clavo by Hewer Text UK Ltd, Edinburgh

Printed and bound in Great Britain by Clays Ltd, Elcograf S.p.A.

Hodder & Stoughton policy is to use papers that are natural, renewable and
recyclable products and made from wood grown in sustainable forests.
The logging and manufacturing processes are expected to conform to the
environmental regulations of the country of origin.

Hodder & Stoughton Limited
Carmelite House
50 Victoria Embankment
London EC4Y 0DZ

www.yellowkitebooks.co.uk

CONTENTS

INTRODUCTION

Hello. My name's Tommy Trotter, and I want to start by giving you a round of applause to welcome you into the next phase of your life. You are about to meet a new version of yourself – someone who is healthy, happy, confident and energised.

I know what you're thinking – *but Tom, why are you clapping for me?! I haven't even bloody done anything yet!*

Well, I'm here to tell you that you *have*. You have opened up this book, which means you have felt a calling in your heart to make some changes and improve your health and fitness. Through the very act of turning to this first page you have demonstrated that you are ready to show up and strap in. And that, my friend, is *highly* commendable. Now that you're here, I can't wait to go on this journey with you. I'll be with you every step of the way.

Perhaps this is the first time you have felt the pull to get fit, or maybe this isn't your first rodeo. You might have tried overhauling your fitness in the past. Perhaps you found it too difficult, or punishing, and you gave up. Maybe it was boring, or stressful, or life got in the way. You made your excuses, you cancelled the gym membership, you told yourself, 'I'll start again next week/month/year', but then never did.

Look, I'm not here to judge. In fact, I completely understand it. If something feels like a chore, why the hell would you want to do it? It's extremely difficult to stay consistent and remain motivated in an activity when you don't feel good at it, you don't enjoy it, and essentially you hate every second of it.

However, I want to show you that there is another way. Just because it hasn't stuck in the past, doesn't mean it won't this time. Not only can fitness be achievable and become a seamless habit in your life, it can also be *exciting* and *fun*. And if you don't believe me right now, I am convinced you will be on board by the time you finish this book. Or your money back! (Sadly, I cannot actually honour this, but it's the thought that counts.)

Given that we're going to be spending a lot of time together on this journey towards joyful health and fitness, I feel that we should probably get to know each other. I'll go first.

You may already know me from my Instagram and TikTok accounts, where I post lots of motivational fitness content with a touch of silliness – particularly the videos featuring my dear old mum, Sally. (Who is definitely more famous than me.) But you might not know what led me here, to writing this book.

It all began on the Isle of Wight, where I was born and raised with my five siblings. You could usually find me running around barefoot on the beach like some sort of feral animal – I always loved moving, and I loved being outdoors. We were raised pretty much single-handedly by my mum (Dad was in the military, and he wasn't around so much) and she was (and still is) the inspiration that fuels so much of what I do. She always taught me that authenticity is the secret to a flourishing, happy life – that if you shine your light, you'll attract the right light to shine right back to you.

I kept this advice in mind when I set out to achieve my dream of becoming a pro rugby player. I had always loved sport, and when I started playing rugby in school I realised I was pretty good at it. One thing about me: once I get something in my head, I'm like a dog with a bone. There is no stopping me. So after I finished my GCSEs, I secured a place at a rugby academy on the mainland (aka England) – essentially a boarding school where they treat you like a proper rugby player to prepare you for becoming a pro, and where you live, breathe and train rugby.

If you're surprised that I was a rugby player, you wouldn't be the only one. I was always the smallest and youngest on the field – little virgin Tommy Trotter playing amongst all these rowdy, beefy lads. It's also true that my eccentric and flamboyant personality didn't exactly fit the stereotypical rugby mould. But keeping in mind my lessons from old Sal, I never shied away from being different – and, in fact, I actively embraced it. I knew that I had to work hard to prove myself, focusing on strength and agility, and I stayed true to myself to earn respect among my teammates. During this time I had to grow up very quickly. I learned the values of leadership, togetherness, teamwork, discipline and the power of working hard to achieve greatness. These values are still extremely important to me.

After playing pro rugby for a couple of years, I realised that it wasn't my destiny after all. Let's be honest: I'm from a big family, so I will go out of my way to be the centre of attention. I started posting fitness videos online during my rugby training just for fun, and I filmed one with my mum where we went for a run together, which went viral. People seemed to enjoy my lighthearted approach to fitness, and I started to think: *Hang on, maybe I can actually make a difference to other people's lives through exercise?* So, at this point I decided to quit pro rugby, and instead travelled the world focusing on content creation and launching my coaching business and app – which is now booming. My mission? Improving as many lives as possible through the power of fitness.

I think the reason why my videos and coaching resonate so much is that I *know* fitness can be intimidating. As much as I've always been 'sporty', I too have felt the pressures of looking a certain way, of worrying whether I'm good enough, of struggling to get up in the morning and wondering what the point is. But I also know that fitness fuels my relentlessly positive attitude. I always say that my morning workout is like mounting a unicorn, to gallop me into a better day. It's not a punishment. It's a beautiful, magical force for good. It reminds me that I can do hard things, which spills out into every area of my life, keeping me motivated and inspired in everything I do. Life can be challenging and uncertain, but fitness grounds me, putting me in the best possible position to make the most out of every circumstance.

You don't need me to tell you the numerous benefits of getting fit, but I'll remind you of a few anyway. Regular exercise can lengthen your life, reduce your risk of serious illness, help you maintain a healthy weight and make you feel happier and more confident. But I know that it can be hard to commit to making these changes. My clients always tell me that they *want* to get fit, they know about all those benefits, but getting up onto that unicorn just feels too difficult. They don't know where to start, they're scared to take the leap and they lack confidence and self-belief. But eventually, with a little bit of help from yours truly, they end up riding off on that unicorn with more speed than they ever thought possible. And with this book you'll also be empowered with the tools to mount your own unicorn. Giddy-up!

My approach works because it's all about kindness, compassion and gradual improvement. It's about creating a safe space, free from judgement and stress. It's not about making big, terrifying changes overnight. It's not about burning out. It's about creating habits that you can *actually* stick to, even when the shit hits the fan. It's about balance – sticking to your workout even after having one too many glasses of wine the night before (and forgiving yourself if you don't manage it).

My mum is living proof of this. Although she has always been active, she has recently decided – in her seventies – that having a consistent fitness routine makes her life better. She knows that health is wealth. She wants to live longer and be stronger for her kids and grandkids. Even though she still works in the NHS, she knows that just committing to a 20-minute strength workout or a

5k run before she heads off to work makes her feel fitter, healthier and happier. She still enjoys socialising and knocking back the vino, so she isn't making any sacrifices – only improvements. She is an inspiration, and a reminder that change is always possible, whatever your age or life circumstances.

So, no matter how scared or unsure you are, you're still *here* – and I'm here with you, as your personal hype-man. I'll provide you with the motivation, accountability, positivity and practical tips to make *this* fitness journey the one that actually sticks. Let me tell you, you *do* deserve that applause. Good golly, I'm so proud of you already.

THE END GOAL

Whatever your unique goals and aims for wanting to get fit, I want to make you a few promises as we embark on this voyage of discovery. As long as you hold up your end of the bargain – sticking to this guide as much as possible and trying your best – you will eventually . . .

- Meet (or surpass) the NHS guidelines for exercise of completing 150 minutes (or 2.5 hours) of moderate intensity exercise each week (the kind that raises your heart rate, but you could still hold a conversation). I know that might seem intimidating, but that's just 20 minutes of exercise per day. This is the minimum recommended amount of exercise for reducing the risk of serious illness later in life, but even more can mean you'll thrive, rather than just survive. (We'll explore the main differences between high-, moderate- and low-intensity exercise on page 77.)
- Have a routine that includes a balanced mix of different types of exercise – from cardio to strength and to low-intensity exercises that boost your flexibility and mobility. Maybe one of

these scares you more than the others, but by the end of my plan I want you to feel comfortable to try different things. You won't just be a one-trick pony (or unicorn).

- Notice that exercise has become a non-negotiable part of your life. It's fun, makes you feel good and you can actually *feel* the benefits. It no longer relies on willpower and is as much a part of your life as showering or brushing your teeth.

- Believe that you have become (or are on the path to becoming) the best version of yourself. The most energised, vibrant, confident version of you, who can't wait to get up every morning – to rise *and* shine.

HERE'S HOW WE'RE GOING TO DO IT

The destination might seem a long way away, but we're going to take the scenic route and enjoy the ride. All aboard! Fasten your seatbelts!

Rather than diving in at the deep end, my plan is all about taking things step by step and levelling up as we go. As you go through the book you'll work through my 7 Levels that will take you from a complete fitness novice to someone who is comfortable and confident with multiple forms of exercise.

I strongly advise that you work through the book in order, as each level has been carefully crafted to help you to up your game from the one before. Each is designed to push you a little further out of your comfort zone – but gently, so it's not a massive shock to the system.

You can spend as much time on each level as you like, but I'd recommend around two weeks per level. In my opinion, this is a good amount of time to get comfortable with the new level, but not too long that you outstay your welcome (no offence). After all, improvement and progress will only come from pushing yourself a little harder as you go along – you can't expect things to change if you always stay the same. By levelling up, you will keep evolving, adapting and showing yourself what you're truly capable of. You'll unlock different layers of yourself that you didn't know existed. And once you have completed my final level – Level 7 – you will have all the mental and physical tools you need to live a happy, healthy life.

In each level, to break the process down into even more manageable chunks we'll work through my Four Fs: FOCUS, FEAR, FITNESS and FUN. Let me explain in a bit more detail what these categories mean.

FOCUS: I'm a massive believer that half the challenge with physical movement is getting your head in the game. For each level, I'll show you how you can focus on what really matters and shift your mindset into the best possible place for a healthy, active lifestyle. Without focus we get distracted, we make excuses, we fall off the wagon. In the focus sections, you'll discover how to find your motivation, build discipline, adapt your diet, track your progress, make use of your community and harness the positive impact so you notice the benefits in the rest of your life. Over the course of the levels you'll notice your mindset becoming more and more positive, optimistic, motivated and energised. Once this mindset is firmly secured, you won't have to keep quitting and starting over. You'll be locked in and focused for the long haul. To infinity, and beyond!

FEAR: There are so many fears that hold us back in life, and especially when it comes to exercising. It's okay to be scared, but it's *not* okay to let your fears get in the way of the life you were destined to lead. I want to show you how you can face your biggest fears – because on the other side of fear, there's freedom. In each level, we'll tackle some of the most common fears and roadblocks to getting fit, dismantling some of the assumptions we make about ourselves and fitness itself. From the negative self-beliefs that stop us exercising, to fears around body image, to preventing and managing injury. You'll learn that fear isn't something to run away from – it's part of the journey, and getting comfortable with discomfort is the secret to making the biggest strides.

FITNESS: This is where we'll get into the nuts and bolts of physical fitness. No more, 'I don't know what I'm doing', because now you will! To begin, I'll show you how you can make movement a habit, before we progress into strength-training moves, how to get into (and improve) your cardio fitness, the importance of low-intensity training and the art of recovery. Once you've worked through each stage, you'll end up completing my 14-day fitness challenge in Level 7, which will pull together everything you've learned. The aim of the game? To give you a well-rounded understanding of fitness, so you feel able to go forth on your own unicorn and choose your own fitness adventure – whether you have a gym membership or prefer to exercise from home.

FUN: You can't spell Tom Trotter without fun (not technically true, but don't think too deeply about it). With that in mind, you'll find a challenge at the end of each level to help you embrace and enjoy every step of the process. From exercise Easter egg hunts and wine-bottle workouts to sports-day games, these challenges will remind you that exercising doesn't have to be so serious, and you'll see that fitness really is the stuff of life.

Now we have got all that housekeeping out of the way, it's time to work through my 7 Levels. So, dust off your trainers, kiss your biceps, draw some stripes on your face (optional) and tell yourself, 'I can bloody do this.'

Let's. F**cking. Go.

THE HARDEST PART IS STARTING

FOCUS: PREPARE YOUR MIND

I have noticed that a lot of people seem to think getting into fitness goes a bit like this:

1. Join a gym.
2. Go to the gym.
3. Keep going to the gym (maybe for a few weeks) until you eventually walk out looking and feeling completely different.
4. Mission complete!

Sadly, this isn't quite how it works. This process doesn't take into account the mental preparation and perseverance needed to actually make long-term, sustainable changes. It assumes that you will keep showing up to the gym, day in and day out, like some sort of robot.

But the reality is, we are not robots. We are products of our thoughts and beliefs, which have the power to make or break our exercise routines. If you believe exercise is something you should just be able to do easily, you'll become deflated when things start to get tough. If you're not clear about *why* you're doing it, you'll struggle to maintain motivation. If you feel bogged down by your past, rather than excited by your future, it'll be way too easy to accept defeat. And so it becomes a vicious cycle, where you give up, then when you try to start again you find you're making all the same mistakes.

I want to help you break this cycle. If you can take the time to sort your mind out *before* you even lace up a pair of trainers, roll out a mat or step foot inside a gym, you're much more likely to set yourself up for greatness. *Your body follows what your mind allows.* Get your mind right, and the rest will become a hell of a lot easier.

Find your 'why'

So many people tell me that the reason they don't maintain a fitness routine is because their motivation drops off a cliff. So let's start there, shall we? What actually *is* motivation?

We often think of motivation as a feeling, or a thing, that we either have or we don't. But that's not really the case. According to the Oxford English Dictionary definition, motivation means 'a reason or reasons for acting or behaving in a particular way'. Basically, the reason *why* you're doing something is what keeps you doing it. This reason is what keeps you feeling motivated.

This is absolutely necessary in all areas of our lives. Our motivations keep us working towards our goals. Why do you want to do well at your job? Because you're motivated to earn money, or help people, or gain recognition – or maybe a mixture of all of the above. Why do you want to save up for a new house and go through all the admin of moving and renovating? Because you're motivated to have a better quality of living for your family. Why do you have a shower every day, without fail? Because you're motivated to be clean and hygienic, so that you don't repel everyone you come across.

Without motivation, we'd get absolutely nothing done. If we don't have a solid reason for doing something, why would we bother?

The problem is, our thoughts about motivation are all wrong when it comes to fitness. We think we should just be instinctively motivated. We think it's some kind of magical state that we either achieve or don't achieve. But, just like in every other area of our lives, we need to be motivated *by something*. We need to have a *reason* (or reasons) for doing it. And this can't be any old reason; your reason is not going to be the same as that of your sister, your mate, or the 6ft 7in personal trainer who works at the gym. It needs to be one that feels overwhelmingly important *to you*.

We all have different reasons for doing the things we do – we have different quirks and incentives that make us tick, and fitness is no different. The trick is to find *your* biggest, overriding, most important reasons, as these will keep you going when the going inevitably gets tough. I call this finding your 'why'.

In my opinion, the 'why' is even more important than the 'what' and the 'how' of exercising. It's the quiet, magical thread that keeps you invested and keeps you *motivated*. Yep, if you've felt like you kept losing motivation in the past, hopefully it all makes sense now. You need to have a really clear vision and reason in order to put your best foot forward.

So, what is your 'why', Tom? Thanks for asking. My why is to put myself in the best possible position to tackle my day, and my life. For me, movement and exercise puts me one step closer to a better day. I love the endorphin rush I feel after. I love that sometimes I might wake up when it's dark and lonely and I'm in a terrible mood, but as soon as I start moving I experience a burst of positivity. It gets me into the saddle on the unicorn of life. I feel that I can conquer anything. That's my biggest why – it makes me feel *empowered*.

I have other whys, too, of course. I want to keep my body fit and healthy so I am able to handle whatever life throws my way.

I want to avoid disease and live with energy and vitality. I want to maintain a healthy weight and like the look of the guy I see in the mirror (there's no shame in that, and we'll come back to that in Level 2). But my biggest overarching why is the way I know that exercise makes me feel – and that's enough to get me up and at it every day.

Your why will probably shift depending on where you are in your life. Also, if you don't know how good exercising feels (yet), you might need something bigger and more long-term to keep you going. One of my clients told me his why was being able to run around playing football with his kids. He wanted to feel like he could play with them for as long as possible. Another client told me that their mum had passed away from heart disease, and her why was wanting to prevent this happening to her, so that she could stick around longer for her loved ones. A friend of mine lacked confidence, and his why was to feel happier in his own skin. My mum's why is to stay happy, well-oiled and live longer. (After all, studies have found that regular physical exercise is associated with an increase in life expectancy of between 0.4 and 6.9 years.[1]) Each one of these people has stuck to their exercise routine because their why is *bloody powerful*.

These particular whys also work so well because they're *internal* and *personal*. Your biggest why should focus on how exercise makes *you* feel, not about what others think of you. I have had clients come to me saying that they want to exercise to fit in with their mates who go to the gym, or they want to make their ex jealous. While these motivations might help as an initial push, they're too flimsy, so they don't last. Because if you do a ton of exercise and you *still* struggle to fit in with your mates, and your ex doesn't seem to care how you're looking, what are you left with? You're likely to lose motivation and wonder why you bothered.

1   https://pmc.ncbi.nlm.nih.gov/articles/PMC3395188/accessed: 11.09.2025

Your why should be sturdy. It should come from within – based only on *you*. This is a why where you can control the outcome. You can't control external factors and other people's opinions, but you can control your own decisions.

TROTTER TASK: HOW TO FIND YOUR WHY

If you're not sure what your why is, follow this step-by-step guide to create a clear motivation.

Get clear on your values. What do you care about most in your life? Is it your health, your kids, your partner, your work? Is it energy, freedom, confidence or peace of mind?

Work out what you're lacking. Do you feel like any of the things you value are challenging you right now? Are you feeling sluggish and fatigued? Do you feel unable to keep up with your kids or at work? Is your current lifestyle out of sync with what you value the most?

Write down multiple whys. Based on what you've just uncovered, jot down multiple reasons to work out. They could be things like: get my confidence back; be present for my family; look after my health for longer.

Write a why mission statement. Tie together your whys – or choose the biggest one – to get clear in one statement. Here are some examples:

'I exercise so that I can be the best parent and partner I can possibly be.'

'I exercise so that I can show up fully in my work and life, with self-assurance and creativity.'

'I exercise to give myself mental clarity and peace of mind, to keep depression and anxiety at bay.'

'I exercise to extend my years in good health, so I can continue doing all the things I love for longer.'

'I exercise to maintain a healthy weight, to enhance my physical health and my confidence.'

Make that statement pop. You can do this in a few different ways. You can write it on a poster and stick it up on your wall. You can set it as your phone background; that way, when your alarm wakes you up for your workout, you're reminded. You can simply repeat it to yourself every time you're about to do some movement.

Now that you have a clear and distinct why, you should begin to feel motivated. If your why truly feels important, and aligns with your values, then the only person you'll let down by not sticking to it is *you*.

Remember: lots of things in life are out of your control. But with this, you are in the driving seat. *You* can commit to your why and keep yourself motivated. It all starts by believing you can.

Imagine your future self

Now you know what you're working towards, it's time to put yourself into the shoes of your future self. How do you want your fitness journey to change you? Who do you hope to become?

Let's do a fun little exercise, shall we? It requires a bit of imagination, so put your fantastical goggles on and let's take a trip into two different kinds of future. Two parallel universes, if you will. The one where you embark on this fitness journey and the one where you don't (or where you give up before you've even picked up speed).

First, let's imagine you continue along your current trajectory. You don't have a fitness routine and you're doing more or less the same things as you're doing now. Besides not moving much, perhaps that also includes not getting enough sleep, eating a lot of junk and just generally not being particularly kind to yourself. What does your life look like?

Be realistic. If you continue along the path you're on, you're likely to feel the same things you're feeling now – and they might even get *worse* over time. You can't expect to change without making changes. Maybe you imagine that your future self has put on more weight. Maybe you're still single, or in the same relationship that makes you unhappy. Maybe you're lacking in ambition and motivation at work. Maybe you're unconfident and unhappy and you feel bad about yourself. Don't let me put words into your own story – I want you to think, realistically, about what your life might look like. *Not* making a choice is still a choice. Is this the life you want to lead? You *can* choose something different.

Next, I want you to picture a different version of yourself. This is the *best* version of yourself you can possibly imagine. Again, be realistic. You're not going to suddenly become an astronaut or run a marathon every day like the Hardest Geezer. But maybe you're up every day with your alarm and feeling excited about the day ahead. Maybe you're a member of a run club, or you play padel, or you walk to work. You're active and full of beans. You enjoy working out and it doesn't feel so hard. Maybe you feel confident at work, you're in a great relationship and you feel comfortable in your friendships. Is this version of you happy and fulfilled? Are you energetic and enthusiastic? This doesn't need to be a pipe-dream. You *can* become this person.

Now, I'm not saying that an exercise routine can solve all your problems, nor is it the *only* thing standing between you and your best self, but I am saying that it's a very good place to start. I'm not a therapist or a psychologist, but I *am* a fitness coach, and I have seen first-hand how exercise has the power to change lives for the better. (I don't want to get ahead of myself here. We'll explore how and why the lessons from exercise can spill out into every area of your life in Level 7.)

For now, I just want you to picture that positive version of yourself and believe that it *is possible to become them.* In fact, screw that; you don't need to *become* them. They already exist, inside of you. It's your choice whether you want to pull them out and allow them to see the light of day. Come on, friend, that version of you deserves to see the daylight.

TROTTER TASK: CREATE A VISION BOARD

If picturing your future self in your mind feels a little difficult, you can make a vision board as a visual representation of everything you want to become. This is something you can actually look at, to remind you of why the hell you're doing this. You can either do this the old-fashioned way with some paper, magazine clippings and glue, or you can pull together a bunch of photos in a Pinterest board or on a collage on your phone that you can look at regularly.

Your vision board will be completely unique to you – it's aligned with your 'why' and the future you want to create. It should feel motivating and inspiring whenever you look at it.

Here are some ideas of what you could include on it:

- Pictures of yourself, when you believe you were at your happiest and most confident (and maybe at your ideal weight . . . but I would focus on the feeling, rather than the aesthetic).

- Pictures of the kind of active lifestyle you could see yourself leading – bike rides through the countryside, an early morning alarm clock, a post-run coffee with a friend.

- Pictures of anything that represents your broader life goals – success at work, finding love, feeling your best.

- Words, phrases and quotes that reflect the future you're working towards. You might find a few little gems as you work through this book.

Remember: This vision board isn't here to remind you of all the things you're not and everything you lack. It's there to inspire you and remind you that this is all *very* achievable.

Choose your tough

I told you that this journey will be achievable and enjoyable, and while I promise that's true, this is also true: it's gonna be tough.

I'm not saying this to scare you, I'm saying it because I will always be honest with you. And I also want you to *embrace the tough*. For some reason, we've been sent the message that life is only good when it's easy. We have apps and online shopping and food delivery services that mean we don't always have to work hard for what we want – we can just click a button and, voilà, a Chinese takeaway is on our doorstep.

Yet the things in life that are truly worth having – the things that give life meaning – always involve a bit of tough. Like getting a good job, having a baby, falling in love, planning a wedding or passing exams. That feeling when you achieve or complete the thing you've worked towards feels so good simply *because* the journey was tough to get there. The most challenging moments are also the most rewarding.

The thing is, *almost everything* is tough in some way. You can choose the easy route in the moment, but that's not necessarily going to be the easy route later down the line. It's tough being successful at work, at the top of your game, because there's more pressure and responsibility, and it's further to fall. But it's tougher to be unemployed or undervalued at work, or unsure about your direction. Which 'tough' would *you* prefer? I know what I would rather choose.

The same goes for exercising. It's tough to get into shape, but it's tougher to be out of shape. It's tough to work on your strength, but it's tougher to deal with falls and ill-health in older age. I know which kind of tough I would prefer. Would you rather it's tough now, or tough later? It might be hard to get there, but the pay-off is worth it.

I was reminded of this not too long ago, when I received the phone call every son dreads. It was my old mum, sounding faint. 'I've been hit by a car,' she said. My heart sank, and I have never bolted out the door so quickly. She had been cycling to her gym class when she was knocked off her bike. I arrived at A&E to the sight of my mum – drowsy and pale but, most importantly, alive. She had been knocked fully unconscious at the scene and had broken her shoulder, but she was *going to be okay.*

Seeing the crack in her helmet from the impact when it hit the concrete, I couldn't have been more grateful that this piece of safety gear saved her life. But the thing that aided her recovery the most? The thing that got her up, back to work and back to workouts within a matter of days? The incredible health and fitness she had built up from putting herself first and prioritising her exercise. She was in the best possible state to handle an injury – both mentally and physically. Of course her fall was tough, and the road to recovery wasn't easy, but it would've been even tougher had she not been so fit in both body and mind.

She chose the short-term tough, to see her through one of the hardest moments. She prepared for the life she didn't know was coming. Now, she's fighting fit and healthier than ever (while still making adjustments for her injured shoulder).

Life is always going to knock us off our feet (and sometimes, off our bikes) – so much of it is unknown and out of our control. But when it's possible to make choices and decisions, it's up to us to make the right ones. It's up to us to choose the path that might feel more difficult in the moment but will actually save us from much worse difficulty in the long run. My inspirational mum is testament to that.

Choose. Your. Tough.

Manage your expectations

Another big reason why people struggle to maintain a good exercise routine is this: their expectations aren't realistic. Once again, we've been sold a lie (*a lie, I tell you!*) that quick fixes are possible. It probably doesn't help that old diet magazines used to promise things like 'six-pack abs in two days' and utter rubbish like that.

The truth is, fitness is a long game. It's an investment. You won't see results immediately, but that doesn't mean nothing is happening. Quietly, slowly, beneath the surface, with every step, every rep and every time you show up when you don't want to, you're making progress. You just have to believe in it.

Set the intention *right now* that you will still celebrate the small wins along the way. Finding a 2k run easier than last time – that's a win. Lifting a slightly heavier weight – that's a win. Not dreading your workout – it's a win, my friend! You don't need to go from 0–100. You can take it step by step. I will keep reminding you of this during each level of the journey, but keep it in your mind as you get started.

Small wins are still wins. And that's a goddamn fact.

FEAR: UNDERSTAND YOUR NEGATIVE SELF-BELIEFS

So now, hopefully, you're shifting your mindset to one that is positive, realistic and motivated. But we still have some very important work to do. We need to overcome what has been making you feel negative, unrealistic and unmotivated to begin with.

We all doubt ourselves, and we all have deeply held beliefs that hold us back from achieving our full potential. And yes, we *all* have them. Even the people you see on social media who look like they have all their shit together. Even the hottest people you've ever seen have insecurities. You just might never find out what they are.

Often, these start when we're really young and they become more and more solid over time as we find evidence to back them up. If you've always thought you're dumb, you're going to find reasons to believe you're dumb. If you've always thought you're annoying, you're going to find reasons to believe you're annoying. It doesn't make these beliefs true, it just means you have allowed them to become your identity, and you use this identity as a stick to beat yourself with. To tell yourself that you're not good enough.

But I'm going to say something groundbreaking here, and you might not be ready for it: your struggles are actually your strengths. And the sooner you realise this, the better.

As a kid, I was quite a late developer. I had a high voice until I was about 18, and I was never the strongest or fastest on the rugby field. But my mum always taught me to celebrate my authenticity, so I thought to myself, 'Right, what do I have that others don't? How can I harness the skillsets I *do* have to improve and grow?' I knew I was enthusiastic and a hard worker, so I took those attributes and I ran with them – literally. I trained hard and took my sport seriously. Most importantly, I didn't try to tone down the person I was. I wasn't much like the other members of my team – I was much more flamboyant and eccentric than you might expect from a rugby player! Rather than dampening these parts of myself, I continued being the over-the-top, energetic person I am because I knew every team needs different characters to play different roles, and I knew it could help with team morale. My enthusiasm and zest for life paid off in multiple ways – I pushed myself more, and I also boosted the team through losses and challenges with jokes and laughs. I didn't need to be the same as everyone else on the team, and in fact my differences are what made me the player I was (and the person I am today). There is power in difference.

If we can overcome our self-doubts and insecurities, and flip them on their heads, we can unlock that galloping fitness unicorn and ride off into the sunset in no time. Yeehaw!

Who are you, really?

If I stood in front of you and asked you this question, what would you say? Maybe you'd tell me about your job or the industry you work in. Maybe you'd define your identity by your role as a partner, a parent or a friend. We have loads of positive identities and beliefs about ourselves that fire us up and keep us on track. However, if you were being *really* honest with me, you'd also tell me about some negative beliefs you hold:

I'm not smart. I'm unattractive. I find it hard to make friends. I lack confidence.

We all have some kind of negative belief that holds us back and makes us feel unworthy and not good enough, but I want you to forgive yourself for thinking these things. You're human, and we live in a world that encourages us to chase perfection. We've been told that anything short of 'perfect' is total crap. So we tell ourselves that we're useless or rubbish. It's okay to think this way sometimes, because we have been conditioned to do that.

However, this negative self-talk ends now. Well, it might not end *right* now, because it can take a while to unlearn these deeply held negative beliefs. But you can choose not to let these negative thought processes dominate your life. They don't rule the roost anymore. No sir, not on my watch!

You have to consciously remind yourself that these negative beliefs are not who you are, and you're not going to keep feeding into them and seeking out evidence to back them up. Instead, you're going to actively *prove them wrong*. You're going to show them who's boss.

In order to do that, let's go through some of the most common negative self-beliefs that can get in the way of exercising. If any of these resonate with you, I want you to read my words a few times over. Maybe cut out this section and stick it somewhere that you can read it again and again. Use it as a reminder that this belief is not helping you. It's not serving you. It's time to watch that belief fly away. It doesn't belong to you anymore.

'I'm not sporty.' This is one I hear from so many of my clients. Laura* is one example. Aged 32, she had struggled to commit to an exercise routine for her whole adult life. She had signed up to the gym, tried running, and could never seem to make anything stick. When we chatted about this in more detail, she told me that she had a big looming fear that she would just never be *good* at exercise. This took me by surprise, because exercise is something anyone can be good at. You don't need to be the fastest or the strongest to do it – you just need to do it. And then, by doing it, you'll *become* faster and stronger. When I pressed her on this, she told me that she always hated sports in school. She was the slowest in every relay race and was always picked last for every team. She felt like people laughed at and looked down on her. As a result, this became a negative self-belief. She associated movement with getting it wrong and not being good enough.

I told her that we're not in school anymore – we're out here in the big game of life. I told her she doesn't need to win races, she doesn't need to be picked for any teams; all she needs to do is the best she can *for herself.* 'It's you versus you,' I told her. As much as I love sports, and this is my background, I know that this is such a common limiting self-belief, and I want to remind you that being sporty isn't a prerequisite for enjoying exercise. You don't need to be sporty for health and happiness. Now, I can proudly say that so many of my clients who are 'not sporty' have got into shape, become fitter than ever, and some of them have even gone on to run marathons and compete in triathlons. You don't need to compete if you don't want to – this might not be a goal you have on your radar. But the point is, *it's possible.* Your past doesn't dictate your future. And you never know, you might just surprise yourself.

'**I'm too old.**' This is where I wheel out my old mum, Sal. She's a prime example that it's *never too late* to pull your bloody trainers on, lift some weights and get into your best health ever. In fact, there's even more reason to do it when you're getting on a bit.

Exercise keeps you well-oiled, which is especially important when those joints become creaky. It builds muscle mass, which tends to weaken as you get older. And cardiovascular fitness protects against tons of illnesses, from diabetes to heart disease to certain cancers. Just because you have never done something before, doesn't mean it's too late. Reframe this and say to yourself: 'I am older and trying something new to improve my health, which is admirable and impressive.' Because, trust me, it really is.

'I'm too out of shape.' This is another barrier that stops people from exercising, when really it should be the reason *to* exercise. Exercising isn't like a secret club for people who are fit and toned, fast and strong. The reason these kinds of people are overrepresented in the fitness community is because *that's what fitness creates*. I know I might be stating the obvious here, but the cycle goes like this: Exercise → You get in shape. It's not like this: Get in shape → Exercise. No one starts at the finish line. You have to begin at your own start line.

I know it might feel like everyone's looking at you in a class or run-club if you're super slow or trailing behind, but I promise you they're not. At the end of the day, everyone is focusing on their own workout – they have their own goals and targets. If they *were* standing around judging other people, then they're just a weirdo – I don't know what else to tell you. It's so important to get out of the mindset that other people are bothered by what level of in-shape you are. It doesn't matter. Other people's opinions are none of your business.

Then there's the fact that every single person has their insecurities. Yes, even that super-jacked guy who seems to be lifting 10 times his bodyweight. He could be wishing he was faster on his feet. Meanwhile, that super-speedy runner on the treadmill might feel insecure about their upper body strength and flexibility. And those people are probably far busier thinking about themselves, the things *they* want to improve, rather than worrying about you. (No offence.)

Remember, it's only you versus you. Keep your head high and focus on your own path.

'I'm not capable.' For some reason, lots of people think they can't exercise because, well, they *just can't*. Usually, this is because people feel like they lack the knowledge and/or the skills to get fit. But here's the thing: if you lack knowledge and skills, you can gain them. You learned to walk, didn't you? You learned to talk, didn't you? You learned how to ride a bike, how to drive, how to do whatever mad skills that your job requires, didn't you? Humans have an incredible capacity to learn shit. You can absolutely learn how to smash a strength session or hold your own in a yoga class. But you won't become capable at something if you never try to begin with.

We'll go into this in more detail in Level 2 – it's all about embracing being a beginner and getting comfortable with any knocks along the way. But for now, I want you to be gone with this defeatist attitude that you 'can't' do something. It's not because you're incapable, it's just because you don't know it yet. And that's why you're here, reading this book.

'People like me won't be accepted into the fitness world.' I've heard this from lots of different people for various reasons – whether they feel like they won't 'fit in' due to their gender, sexuality, race, disability, class or even just personality traits. And maybe, in the past, that might have been the case. But exercising is so much more accessible and inclusive now – and there are so many options. You can work out at home or you can join clubs to find your own sense of community. And if it doesn't feel welcoming in the particular gym you've signed up to, it might just be the wrong place.

There's no one type of 'fit' person. When we think about the kinds of people who work out, a certain image might come to mind: someone with enormous muscles, who only owns tank tops, who can't think or talk about anything else except for gains and macros. It's *simply not true*. You can be anything you want to be – a comic book fanatic or someone who dresses as an adult baby (I don't judge) and *still* make the choice to get fit. You can be slow or weak or out of shape and *still* make the choice to get fit. Just like I did in my rugby days, you can choose to see those quirks as strengths and wear your differences with pride. I promise you, whoever you are, that exercise is *for* you. You belong here.

Rewrite your story

Whatever identity you have given yourself, whatever negative belief you have inflicted upon yourself – you have the power to change it. You can tell yourself a new story. But you might have to do it a few times before it really sinks in.

Every time you catch yourself saying (or thinking) 'I'm not capable', can you instead say (or think) 'I am capable. I can do this'?

Instead of 'I'm not sporty', can you say, 'I don't need to be sporty to take control of my health'?

Instead of 'I'm too old', can you say, 'I'm making healthy choices – just in time'?

Instead of 'I'm too out of shape', can you say, 'I'm getting into shape'?

Instead of, 'People like me won't be accepted into the fitness world', can you say, 'I deserve to get fit, just like everybody else'?

Sometimes it really is that simple – if you speak that positivity into existence, your mind will start to believe it. Repeat these phrases in the mirror, write them down, put them in a song, do a little dance ... do whatever you need to do to get them into your brain. Give yourself a positive narrative and you can start this journey in the best possible headspace.

FITNESS: INTRODUCING MOVEMENT

I told you that I wouldn't chuck you in at the deep end, and I meant it! In fact, we're going to start in the paddling pool. All you need to do is dip in your toes and you'll begin to realise how good it feels, so you'll *want* to go off into the deep end and have a swim around. But for now, hold your horses (unicorns), because we're gonna get comfortable in the shallow water first.

In my opinion, it's so important to get comfortable with the basics before you overhaul your fitness routine. And what do I mean by 'the basics'? I mean, it's as simple as *moving your body*. Yes, you heard me right. Simply moving. I know this might sound obvious, but the reality is that many of us aren't moving our bodies nearly enough. We work at desks, we drive everywhere, we sit down for dinner and then we sit down in front of the TV. Unless you have a job that involves physical labour or a dog that needs walking otherwise it will run around the house like a lunatic, it's likely that you're not moving enough in your everyday life. And, in my opinion, simple movement is the gateway to structured exercise.

You might be thinking: *But Tom, I know how to move my body. This step is boring. Let me skip it, please!!*

I hear you, comrade. I myself am partial to a more heart-thumping workout than simply walking around the block. However, the walk around the block allows you to do just 1 per cent more than you were doing yesterday. It allows you to get comfortable in your body, to show it what movement can do for it. It dusts off the cobwebs. It allows you to fine-tune where you're at. It allows you to prepare your body and mind for the heart-thumping stuff. So I implore you not to skip this step.

Start by shifting your mindset towards gratitude for being able to move your body at all. You know that feeling when you've stubbed your toe and walking really hurts? You think to yourself, *goddamnit – I wish I appreciated how good it felt to walk on a normal toe!* Then when it recovers it feels amazing, but you quickly forget and take it for granted again. I want you to make a really conscious effort to imagine what life might feel like if you had a stubbed toe, and how nice it is to walk free from pain, free from discomfort. That, my friend, is a gigantic privilege, and it's high time you treated it as such.

Next up, I want you to think about the moments in your day where you're probably cutting corners. Are you getting the lift to go up one floor when you could be taking the stairs? Are you driving to pick the kids up from school when you could walk? Where are there possibilities for movement that you're *not* taking currently?

I'll give you an example. One of my clients is a postman – let's call him Pat. Postman Pat complained that his job involved being sat down in his van all day, and he felt intimidated by the gym and traditional exercise. I suggested he start small. Could he, just once a day, take the stairs to deliver mail in a block of flats, rather than taking the lift? He started doing this, and he told me how out of breath and out of shape he felt. But he kept going, until eventually he was taking the stairs in most of the blocks he was delivering to. After a few weeks, these stairs were no longer making him feel so unfit – his cardiovascular fitness had improved drastically – so he was ready to move on to more intense fitness. This simple change made the world of difference. I'm sure you can find moments in your day to do the same.

Here are a few suggestions to add more movement into your day:

Get your 10,000 steps. Walking is the easiest way to get more comfortable with movement. You can go with friends, take a pet, buy a coffee, listen to a podcast. If it helps you, buy a fitness tracker and compete with yourself to get as many steps into your day as possible (we'll come back to fitness trackers on page 118). You can walk during your lunch break at work instead of eating at your desk. You can walk to and from the station rather than driving. You can *still* walk if it's pissing down with rain – just wear the right shoes and pack a waterproof. There's really no excuse *not* to walk whenever you have the opportunity.

Dust off your bike. You know that two-wheeled thing with a seat and handlebars that has been collecting dust in your shed? That's a bike! It can be used for transportation, but it also is a great form of exercise, so you'll kill two birds with one stone (but please try not to kill any birds while on the bike). Just remember to ride safely – *always* wear a helmet.

Take the stairs. Anywhere – that's the stairs at your office, in your home or apartment building or in the train station. Just like Postman Pat discovered, taking the stairs instead of opting for the quicker route is an easy way to help you build your fitness. It enhances cardiovascular health, improves endurance and muscle strength, and can help you burn off calories. Stair-climbing is not to be sniffed at.

Stand whenever possible. If your working day is mostly spent at a desk, purposely stand on the train or bus during your commute (even when there's a seat available). Even simply standing up without moving a muscle is good for you, as it helps you burn more calories, improves circulation and can reduce the risk of heart disease and diabetes. Aim to stand up once every hour. Another way to do this is to buy a standing desk so you can stand up while working from home.

Make strength building part of your day. Walk with your shopping bags to the car/home – sure, you *could* just put them into a trolley, but that would be far too easy. Carrying your shopping (provided it's just heavy enough to feel like a challenge and not so heavy that it's impossible) is such an easy everyday way to build strength – and also improve balance. There are plenty of things you can make the effort to carry in your everyday life – the laundry basket, your kids, your pets. Anything and everything can become a dumbbell (just make sure you ask for consent if it's another human!).

Stretch it out. Raising your arms above your head for a full-body stretch while you yawn? Yep, that's movement! We'll cover stretching in more detail in Level 4, but for now I want you to simply stretch in ways that feel good to you – whether you're cooking dinner, sitting at a desk or about to get into bed at night. Notice how good it feels in your muscles, tendons and ligaments when you roll your shoulders, lift your torso, rotat·e your ankles? See? Movement is enjoyable. You're beginning to get the hang of it now.

FUN: YOUR DAILY MOVEMENT EASTER EGG HUNT

Who doesn't love a good Easter egg hunt? Except with my version, you're searching for moments of movement in your everyday life, and instead of chocolate, the reward is setting yourself on a path of healthy living.The aim of the game? Do five of these exercise eggs every day to win.

Why? They're short, they're sweet and they add up. They're easy to find, so you can add exercise into your day without fuss or drama. When you add exercise into the things you're *already* doing, that's when you create a habit.

How many players? You can do it by yourself (you versus you, baby!) or you can get your family and friends involved for a little bit of healthy competition.

What's the prize? Shiny gold glory. (But if you want to give yourself a bit of chocolate once you complete all of these, go for it – you've earned it!)

Shampoo shoulder curls. While you lather your shampoo or conditioner, do 10 big shoulder rolls backwards, then 10 big shoulder rolls forward.

Calf raises while you brush your teeth. Simply lift your heels off the floor, rising onto the balls of your feet. Pause at the top, squeezing your calf muscles, then lower your heels back down. Keep going for as long as you're brushing your teeth.

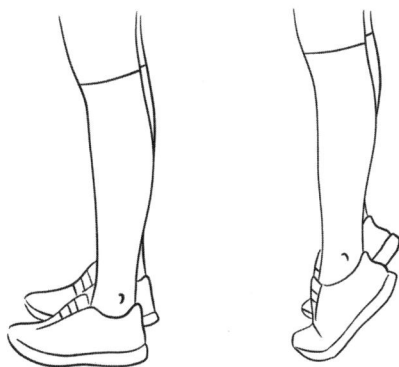

Coffee lunges. While you're waiting for your coffee (or tea) to brew, do some simple lunges in the kitchen. Simply step one leg forward, then bend both knees while keeping your upper body upright. Hold, then switch.

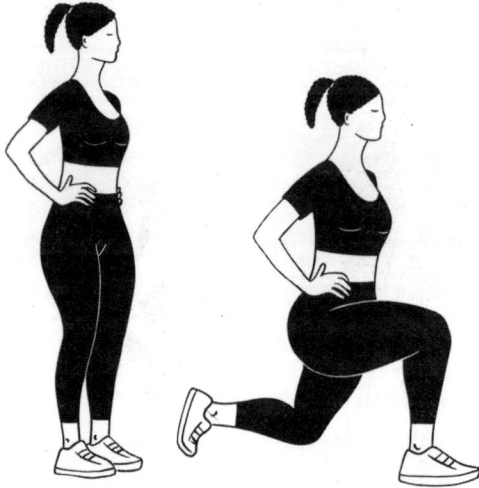

Change your transportation. Can you get to work by bike or on foot? This counts as an egg, my friend!

Walk 'n' talk. Walk around every time you need to take a phone call. Or – bonus – walk with a colleague in your lunch break. See if you can hit 4,000 steps in one go.

Skip the lifts. Take the stairs in your office or place of work.

Miss your stop. Get off your train or bus one stop early (or one stop late) and walk a little longer.

Bicep bag carrying. No asking for help. No taking the trolley. Just you, your guns and shopping bags filled with groceries. Bonus egg if you can lift them for a little bicep curl.

Squat 'n' tidy. Every time you pick up something off the floor, do a squat. (And if you're getting down on the floor, try to get up without using your hands to help you.)

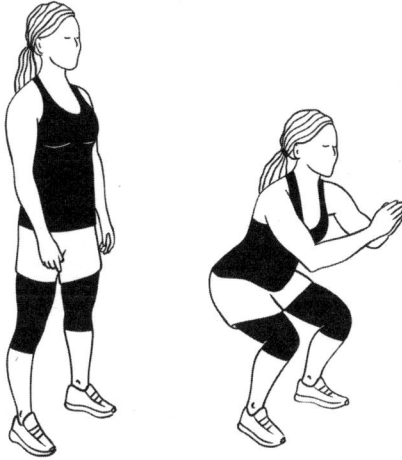

Vacuum 'n' engage. Each time you push out that vacuum cleaner, engage your arm muscles and your core.

TV ad-break planks. Make that ad break feel productive; try to hold a plank until the show starts again. Lie on the floor with your forearms on the ground, directly under your shoulders. Tuck in your toes and lift your knees so your body is in a straight line from your head to your heels. Hold on to this position for as long as possible – ideally until the end of the ad break, but if you only manage one ad at first, that's good enough!

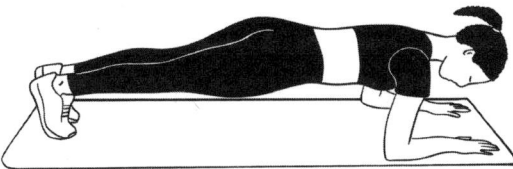

Go-to-bed dance party. When you're getting into your pyjamas, brushing your teeth, doing your skincare and whatever else, put on your favourite song and dance along. Let yourself wiggle and be free!

Remember, every time you choose to do these actions, you are choosing yourself!

FIND YOUR RHYTHM

FOCUS: CREATE A ROUTINE

In Level 1 you learned all about finding your motivation – the long-term 'why' that will act as a guiding force throughout this whole journey. But I'll be really honest with you: motivation is not enough to stay committed and see results. Your motivation will come and go, and there will be days where you'll think about your why and then decide, 'I actually don't really care about that today. I just want to stay in bed.' And in times like this, you need to fall back on discipline.

I know the word 'discipline' has negative connotations, but in the context of exercise, discipline is about empowerment – it's *sticking to your own rules*. It's about showing up and doing the damn thing, even when your motivation is off on holiday somewhere. It's about creating a structure and routine that you can easily stick to, so you don't have to rely so strongly on your motivation day to day. It's about creating the right environment to put your why into action.

At this early stage, you don't need to have a solid five-day routine. You don't need to wake up at the crack of dawn to exercise. You don't need to join a gym. Hopefully, you're already building a habit of incorporating more movement into your day, and now is the time when we start implementing a bit more structure. But we can still keep it light and manageable, and increase it gradually as we go along. Think of yourself as an exercise gardener: you've just got to plant the seeds of new habits and allow them to grow.

NOTE: When we talk about building a routine and creating a structure in this section, you still might be thinking – *wtf, I still don't know what kinds of exercise I'm doing yet!* That's totally okay. This section is just to get you thinking about preparation, and carving out time in your schedule for fitness, while removing any potential excuses that could stand in your way. You can fill in the blanks as you progress through the book and learn more about different kinds of workouts, so you know what you're doing in the space you've created. For now, it's okay to view this as your 'planning' phase. Get those cogs turning!

Create a clear structure

I'm sure you already have a routine in your day that you feel super comfortable with. You wake up at the same time for work, have a shower, brush your teeth, have your same old breakfast and listen to the same podcast on the way home. We're creatures of habit, after all, and routine can feel like a safety net. When I travelled for a long time, around Australia and south-east Asia, one of the things I struggled with the most was a lack of routine. As exciting as travelling is, consistency is the thing we tend to miss after long stretches of time, because that regular rhythm is comfortable and peaceful. Now, I always try to make some kind of routine wherever I go, because it feels like a comfort zone that reminds me of home.

Introducing fitness into your life can feel like the biggest push outside of your regular comfort zone. But here's the thing about routine – once you create it, and you get used to it, *then* it becomes comfortable. Once you have an exercise routine that you enjoy, that works for you and feels good, it can become that safe space for you. It might not feel that way at first, but I promise that if you stick at it it'll become just as non-negotiable as doing a number two, and just as enjoyable as your first bite of dinner every night. Get your routine nailed and it'll become second nature.

I've said this before and I'll say it again: you are in the driver's seat of your life. When it comes to creating your exercise routine, you are in control. What works for me might not work for you. I think, in the fitness world, there's a lot of pressure to do fitness a *certain way*. There's a lot of emphasis on getting up while it's still dark, shoving your head in a bowl of ice and then punishing yourself for an hour in the twilight before you are allowed to go about your day. If you want to do it like this, *great*, but I'll guess that for the average person this just seems a tad intense, if not entirely impossible.

Let me tell you something clearly: you don't need to wake up at the crack of dawn. You don't need to do hour-long workouts every day. You really don't need to shove your head into a bowl of ice (although it does actually feel quite nice, so if you want to, go for it!). You can slot in your workouts when it works best for you. Your logistics matter. That influencer online? They don't lead the same lifestyle as you – whether that's a demanding office job or caring for kids and elderly parents – so their workout regime won't be the same as yours. First and foremost, let go of that comparison. Your routine is *yours* and yours alone. It doesn't matter when you do it or where you do it, it just matters that you're doing the damn thing, and you're doing it consistently.

Consistency = progress.

TROTTER TASK: CREATE YOUR STRUCTURE

Create space. First of all, I want you to have a look at your calendar or planner. Go on, do it right now. Where do you tend to have chunks of free time? I'm not talking about an entire morning or entire afternoon, it could just be 20 minutes. Can you take longer lunch breaks when you're working from home? Do you have some time in the evenings, after your kids have gone to bed, or perhaps in the mornings before they wake up? Maybe some days in your week are chocka, but you have more free time on Wednesdays, Saturdays and Sundays when work is quieter, or when grandparents are over to help out with the kids. Wherever you see these free blocks, schedule in a workout. You don't need to know what you're doing during each of these sessions yet – for now, just put aside the time. It's all about setting the intention. You're saying: *This is my time to move.*

SEPTEMBER						
MON	TUE	WED	THU	FRI	SAT	SUN
1	2 GYM	3 OFFICE	4	5	6 SWIM	7
8 OFFICE	9 GYM	10	11	12 PUB	13	14
15	16	17	18 GYM	19	20 SWIM	21
22	23 OFFICE	24	25 GYM	26	27 PUB	28
29	30					

Sprinkle, then pour. Please, don't go gung-ho with your workouts at this stage. If you have a whole hour free on a Friday afternoon, I'd still recommend you just block out 20 minutes for a quick session. Eventually, you can build it up into something longer, but I'd suggest sprinkling smaller workouts throughout your week so it feels more manageable. Then once you have built the habit, you can start extending and adding on. For complete beginners: it could be worth starting with just one exercise session in a week. Then after two weeks, add another, and after three weeks, add another. You get to do this at your own pace. Remember, you're the driver and you're controlling the speed. Keep it manageable, and you're more likely to stick to it.

Schedule realistic rest days. Let's say you have all of Sunday free, it could be tempting to block this out as a hardcore work-out day. But let's be realistic, you might have children at home and no childcare, or you might want to spend a full day with your family without needing to escape to the gym, or you might just want to mooch around going for coffee or seeing friends. Your exercise routine shouldn't compromise your lifestyle – you still deserve to have a nice time. In Level 6, we'll discuss how you can *combine* your social life with exercising, but for now, it's okay to prioritise both separately. Don't overload your schedule – make sure you have time for both.

Experiment and make changes. As you progress through this book you'll learn about the different types of exercise you can do to fill these slots. Maybe you'll do strength workouts on Mondays and Wednesdays, go running on Fridays or do Pilates on Sundays. Perhaps some of these sessions are in the gym near your office, while others are at home. Come up with a structure that is achievable and works for you, but it's okay to keep changing it. If that lunchtime run on a Friday is proving too difficult with the amount of work you have on, could you

> run on the weekend instead? If something feels too tight and hard to fit in, that doesn't mean you should stop altogether, it just means you need to adapt your routine and give it a refresh. Once you make it, it's not fully set in stone. You can keep returning to it, tweaking and swapping.
>
> **Commit for 8 weeks.** Once you have found a routine that you're really enjoying and seems to work well, I'd recommend sticking to it (as much as possible) for eight solid weeks. For me, this is the amount of time it takes for a routine to bed in and become really comfortable so that I can almost do it on autopilot, same as putting the kettle on after lunch. I also think two months is the best amount of time in which you can see progress and results.

Set yourself up for success

Once you have carved out that time and energy for your workouts, it's important to give yourself the best possible environment to make it happen. If you fail to prepare, you should prepare to fail.

You wouldn't rock up to a supermarket with no idea what you need to buy, then just wander around aimlessly. I mean, maybe you would, but that's not very productive, is it? You're likely to forget the things you actually need and come home with a load of unnecessary crap. It's always a better idea to go shopping with a list. And the same goes for exercise. If you're ready for your workouts, it's much easier to stick to them. Remove any potential barriers in your way like a titan and you'll set yourself up for greatness.

Here are my five golden rules of prep for getting your workout walloped:

1. **Secure the kit.** You don't need tons of fancy equipment to start exercising. I'd recommend starting off with a good pair of running trainers (which you can also wear for gym/strength exercises), an exercise mat and some sweat-wicking garms (sports bra, t-shirt, leggings, shorts, etc.). You don't need particularly expensive items, just what feels comfortable and won't fall apart quickly. However, I would also recommend you buy things that you like the look of, so you get excited to put them on and strut into your workout.

2. **Make sure your kit is ready the night before.** Whether you work out in the mornings or evenings, it always helps to have everything laid out so that you can change into it as soon as you're ready to get moving. You don't want to hold yourself back by rummaging through your drawers hunting for socks, or realising your leggings are in the wash.

3. **Always have a plan.** It's no good getting your kit out, putting it on and then going, 'ummm, what kind of exercise shall I do today?' Have a plan in your mind for what you want to do; maybe that's a short run, maybe a leg or ab day, or perhaps it's a Pilates session or a swim at the local pool. Within that, make sure you know if you're following along with one of the workouts in this book, with a YouTube video, or doing a certain amount of reps of each of your favourite moves. Save all your favourite routines in an easy-to-access folder. This means that you can show up and get started without having to think too deeply about it. You have already laid the groundwork, all you have to do is follow along.

4. **Visualise yourself doing your workout.** I know a lot of people say you should visualise how you will feel *after* your workout, and yes, that's great, but I would also recommend that when your alarm goes off and you can't be bothered and you really just want

to hit snooze, imagine yourself *doing* your workout. Visualise yourself picking up those dumbbells or pounding the pavement, or whatever it is you're doing that day. Picture your mind and body flooding with endorphins, the pride you feel from going up a weight bracket, the smugness at bloody showing up, the sweat that only comes from working hard. Imagine yourself doing it, and it's like you're already there – all you have to do is remove it from your head and place it into reality. Easy peasy.

5. **Have a backup ready**. Whatever workout you've planned, have an easier version in your mind locked, loaded and ready to go. This means that if you're feeling hungover, exhausted or just don't have enough time, you'll still do *something*, rather than skipping it altogether. Say you have planned a 5k run, can you just do 2k? Say you have planned a 30-minute strength session, can you just do 15 minutes? In all likelihood, you'll get started and think – *actually, I can go on for a bit longer or a bit further.* And then you'll end up doing the workout you originally planned. But if you don't, that's totally fine too. Sometimes we need to take it a little easier and give ourselves a break. Trust your mind and body.

Allow for flexibility

It might seem like a contradiction to say have a structure but also stay flexible, but in my opinion, having a solid structure in place is *necessary* to allow you to deviate, because it means that even if you switch it up and change things around, you still always have a solid base to come back to, your safe space.

Life happens, and sometimes getting a workout done is just not possible. Maybe you're sick or injured, perhaps you're working 14-hour days and barely have time to eat, let alone move. Forgive yourself for these moments, and remember that they will pass. Make the relevant adjustments and go back to Level 1 if you need to. Just because you don't have time for a proper workout, could you walk and talk in a meeting with a colleague? Could you squeeze in a stretch before bed? However busy you are, there are always ways to move – just a little – in your day. And in my opinion, even these small bursts of movement can make a difference to whatever you're dealing with. It gives you some time just for *you*, and there ain't nothin' more important than that.

Excuses, be gone!

Here are some important reminders when you feel yourself reaching for the same old excuses:

'I'm too busy.' If you're working a lot and spinning a lot of plates, I commend you. You're doing so well, and you should be proud of that. But I would also ask you to be super realistic and harsh with yourself – do you struggle to find time to exercise but can find 10 minutes to mindlessly scroll through social media or watch random YouTube videos? I'm not saying you *can't* do these things anymore, but I'd ask you to consider what you're giving your free time to – particularly activities that are not benefiting you. Could you, every other day, swap that time with some exercise – even if it's only 10 minutes. It all adds up. You might even find that you then feel more capable to tackle whatever you have on – exercising enhances focus and improves mood, which could be exactly what you need to get through your busy day, week or month . . . or even your year.

'I'm too tired.' Oh, I hear you! Sometimes you feel like you can barely lift your head off your pillow, let alone rip up those biceps with some dumbbell curls. That said, the thing about exercise is that it *gives* energy. It increases blood flow and endorphins, which can help you feel revitalised and ready to tackle your day. The exact reason why you *don't* want to exercise is the reason why you should. Start off slow, and you can up the ante once you notice your energy improving.

'**I don't feel strong enough today.**' Sometimes your body just ain't feeling it – maybe you're recovering from illness or you're in a particular phase of your menstrual cycle (if you have those). But here's the thing: it doesn't matter. We're not in the business of breaking records (not yet, anyway). Just showing up is enough – even if you're lifting lighter than you did yesterday or running slower than you did last week. Strength is such a mental battle anyway, and the more you can push through those limiting thoughts, the stronger you realise you *actually* are.

Come back to this section whenever you feel your discipline waning. Whenever you feel those excuses creeping in. Forgive yourself, tweak your schedule, and get your head back in the game. You've got this.

FEAR: HOW YOU LOOK IS ONLY ONE PART OF THE STORY

In Level 1 we tackled some of the biggest reasons why people decide to exercise. One of which is that people want to change the way they look. Now, I want to give this reason my full attention because, jeepers creepers, it's a loaded one. And I know it's a big concern for a lot of my clients.

First of all, it's absolutely natural to care about the way you look. Your body is the shell you put out into the world – it's the first piece of information that people gain about us. We live in our bodies day in, day out – we can't get rid of them. And if we don't like the look of the body we're in, this can massively affect our mental headspace and confidence. So if you decide to make changes and adopt a healthier lifestyle because you want to feel better in your own skin, I absolutely commend your courage.

However, I want to show you that how you look is only one part of the story. I want you to view a change in appearance as a happy bonus, rather than the whole goal. Because I know how damaging it can be when a preoccupation with looks goes too far and can actually leave you unhealthier than before. I know, because I've been there.

Aesthetics aren't all they're cracked up to be

Once I finished playing rugby and started doing social media, my exercise goals changed. For such a long time I had been focused on my sport – it had all been about performing to the best of my physical ability, and how fitness made me look was almost irrelevant. However, with rugby life in the rearview mirror, I needed a new goal.

There was a combination of reasons why I started to lose a *lot of weight.* I was travelling around beautiful places, spending a lot of time on the beach, and it was a real ego boost when people noticed my training and how lean I was getting. Then there was the fact that my social media account was growing, which was very image-focused. It felt like the appearance of my body was becoming my identity, and I wanted to make sure I kept it that way.

Remember I told you how I am like a dog with a bone when I get something in my head? Well, being the 'lean muscley guy' became my new chew toy. I never seemed to reach an 'ideal' body, because I just kept pushing my limits even further. Every time I achieved something, it became a new standard that I wanted to beat. Training hard while being in a calorie deficit (burning more calories than I was eating) became my new normal. I should have known how unhealthy this was at the time, but it spiralled out of control.

At the same time, I was still receiving compliments for how I looked. There was definitely an ego thing. People would say, 'wow, that guy is shredded', and I wore it with pride. But what they didn't know is that I had lost my sex drive, I wasn't eating enough and didn't enjoy food anymore, I had barely any social life and I was always knackered. I wasn't just losing muscle mass, I was losing my energy and my spark. I had become so obsessed with how I looked that I had slipped into a mental health condition called body dysmorphia without even realising.

I don't know if there was one specific moment when I noticed I had taken things too far. I do know that some of my family and friends were worried about me, but I had to realise it myself before I could make changes. Now, when I look back at pictures of myself at that time I can see that I look like skin and bone, but I had no idea at the time.

You know what they say: beauty is in the eye of the beholder. And it's really true – in the sense that it's completely subjective. Many people would've thought I looked fucking fantastic when really I was miserable and slipping into dangerous territory. We all perceive looks totally differently, and in fact our own minds can even change when it comes to looks. This is why chasing aesthetics is a losing battle. It's based way too much on perception, and our own perceptions get it completely wrong sometimes.

In my own time, I increased my calorie intake and I scaled back on the obsessive levels of training that I was doing. I learned to prioritise balance over burnout – this is one of my mantras that we will come back to a lot throughout this book. Essentially, it means you don't have to do things to extremes to feel benefits. And in fact, pushing yourself to the limit is *not* the way to go. I still care about the way I look. I like to feel jacked and I get a lot of validation when people think I look good (sorry, not sorry). I'm human, after all.

But I know that getting a 'good body' is never worth the expense of losing my energy, and, let's face it, my soul. I know that how I look is only a small part of the puzzle – the other stuff is so much more important.

Feeling good trumps looking good, every damn time.

Beauty standards: it's a trap!

It makes sense that we all care a lot about how we look. We have basically been trained to care through years and years of watching TV, reading magazines and seeing adverts all full of beautiful people. The idea that looking good = a healthy, happy life is basically considered a fact. However, I have learned from my years in the fitness industry that the people with the most stereotypically 'great' bodies still have their insecurities, and they have made a lot of sacrifices to get there. Perhaps they've sacrificed a social life, and they have no confidence in their intelligence or abilities. Looking a certain way doesn't automatically solve all your problems, in fact, it can create new ones. That's what happened for me.

If you want to change how you look, that's fine, but I want you to keep a few things in mind as you embark on this journey. First, the 'ideal' body is always changing. For men, sometimes it's lean and sometimes it's bulky. I remember the days when, for a man, having a good body was about filling every inch of your tight Topman t-shirt! For women, sometimes you're praised if you're stick-thin, and sometimes it's all about a big bum and big thighs. Why does this happen? Well, it's because there's no one single idea of beauty. It changes depending on culture and trends. And when it comes to your body, the last thing you want to do is chase trends, because they're fleeting – they change just as quickly as they arrived. Instead, I'd ask you to think about an ideal weight or look *for you*. This isn't based on how anyone else looks. It's *you versus you*.

And anyway, trying to look like other people is always going to be impossible. We all have different resources, priorities and requirements – the people you see on Instagram with banging bodies probably have a level of time and access to fitness and healthy food that the average person doesn't. Not only that, there's a very strong chance that they're editing some of their pictures (I have never done this – however, I know that some people do!).

Then there's the fact that we all have completely different body shapes. Some people seem to have pronounced abs without even doing so much as a crunch; they're simply born with it. Some people carry more weight around their thighs, while others carry more in their arms. If I put on any weight, you can always see it in my face – I turn into Mr Chubby Cheeks! Some people have hormonal conditions and genetic predispositions that means they can either see results quickly or very slowly. Because of this, we all respond differently to training. Even if you do the exact same routine as another person, it still won't result in the same body. Once you make peace with that, you can begin to love the body you're in – and learn to track your progress against *yourself*, not against other people.

Comparison is the thief of joy. Another saying that people use all the time, but it's so friggin' true. You really can't compare yourself to others in this big ol' confusing life. You're the only person who is exactly like you; with all your incredible skills, your bangin' personality and the body you live in. Learning to accept and embrace *all of it*, even the parts you don't like so much, is an essential stepping stone on your exercise journey. Your body doesn't just deserve to be loved and accepted once you reach your 'ideal weight' or aesthetic. Our bodies are bloody brilliant, and they deserve our respect – whatever stage we're at.

> **TROTTER TASK: PRACTISE BODY ACCEPTANCE**
>
> I want you to appreciate your body for what it can do, rather than solely what it looks like. I want you to . . .
>
> Look in the mirror each morning and tell yourself, 'This is my body – and it's more than enough.'
>
> Say 'thank you' to your body after all your workouts. Your body helped you run down the street, lift those weights and move freely. It's bloody incredible! Show it some gratitude.
>
> Avoid social media accounts that trigger comparison about your body, and follow accounts that uplift and motivate you.
>
> Speak kindly towards your body – imagine you're speaking to yourself like you'd speak to a friend. You would be kind and positive rather than critical and harsh. We are what we think, so if you force yourself to only think nice thoughts about your body, you will eventually believe them.

Confidence comes from within

I once had a client called Priya* who came to me because her ex had just broken up with her. 'I need a revenge body,' she said. Throughout her relationship she had felt insecure about her weight and her ex often made snide remarks about how much she was eating or whether she'd be able to fit into her jeans. All of this had pushed her self-confidence off a cliff. Still, she loved and missed him, so she thought reaching her ideal weight would show him what he was missing and he'd come crawling back to her.

After a few months of working with me, Priya began to find a renewed love for her body. But it wasn't in the way she expected. She discovered that she loved strength-training (we'll come onto this shortly), because it made her feel powerful and strong. She started attending classes and she found a community that reassured her and made her feel great about herself. Little by little, her confidence grew.

Her body changed, too, and she began to like what she saw in the mirror. But it was self-trust from discipline, empowerment from building strength and a general improvement in her health and fitness that made all the difference. And yes, her ex did come crawling back, sliding into her DMs saying she looked good in one of her pictures. But guess what? Priya had enough self-worth to know she was far too good for him anyway, and she deserved so much better.

Priya isn't my only client who has gone on this kind of journey. Often, looks are the trigger – but it's the inner confidence that becomes much more noticeable. Although her body did change in appearance, she hadn't even reached her 'ideal weight' before she felt *so* much happier and sexier. It's a lesson that true confidence comes from within, *and then* it radiates outwards. The better you feel inside, the better you're going to look. Exercise creates a sense of empowerment and self-belief and gives you a glow that is psychological as much as it is physical.

Your looks are only a small part of who you are. They tell *a* story, but it's not the whole story. Your appearance lives alongside all the amazing qualities you have, that other people would kill for. Your kindness, your empathy, your intelligence, your humour, your enthusiasm and your energy. By the end of this book, I want you to love who you see in the mirror – not because your hips are a certain size or your biceps are defined, but because you *feel* the best you ever have, deep inside.

Exercise Aesthetics: Myths & Facts

MYTH: *Women will get bulky if they lift weights.*
FACT: That female bodybuilder physique you sometimes see? That doesn't come from solely lifting weights, that comes from a highly specific training regime. For the average gal, strength-training isn't gonna make you 'bulky', because testosterone is what plays a huge role in creating those big muscles. For women, strength-training is brilliant for improving strength (duh), bone density, metabolism and muscle tone. It also supports cardio exercise, which can help with weight loss (but we'll come back to that in more detail in Level 4).

MYTH: *Men will become skinny if they run.*
FACT: Yes, cardio is great for weight loss, if that's what you're after. But it doesn't automatically shrink muscle (unless you're running in a calorie deficit – meaning you're not eating enough). If you run or do cardio alongside proper nutrition and strength-training, you will actually enhance muscle definition and tone.

MYTH: *Crunches or ab workouts will give you a flat stomach.*
FACT: Sadly, this isn't quite how it works (as much as I wish it was). You can't target fat loss in one area by exercising that body part. Weight loss comes from overall exercise and diet. However, working your core and abs *will* strengthen and define the muscle beneath any fat storage.

MYTH: *Exercise will 'fix' your body shape.*
FACT: Yes, you can absolutely change your body composition (the ratio of muscle to fat), but what you cannot change is your limb lengths, bone structure and genetic fat distribution. Sadly, I learned the hard way that exercise wasn't gonna make me any taller. Exercise can sculpt within the blueprint that you

already have – and good golly, it's a wonderful blueprint, because it's *yours*.

FITNESS: GAIN STRENGTH

We have touched on strength-training quite a lot over the last few pages, so now it's time to put strength into action. Don't worry, we'll start nice and light and easy (using only body weight), then we'll work up to some more advanced moves, using weights and machines in Level 5.

Why strength-train?

I won't lie to you, there's something a bit caveman about strength-training. It's almost primal to feel a sense of satisfaction and pride when you lift something heavy. Maybe because, back then, you would've needed strength to throw rocks around to keep predators out of your cave. Who knows? But that's how it feels.

I love the feeling of accomplishment that comes from strength-training. It's so easy to measure your progress – not just by the feeling of your muscles popping out of your skin, but by noticing that weights become easier and easier, and you have to start lifting heavier and heavier to feel the challenge.

Strength-training is important for everyone, not just men who want to get hench. It increases your strength, which supports you in every aspect of life – from carrying shopping to doing laundry to looking after kids. It improves bone density, too, which is even more important as you get older and your bones become more brittle. It improves blood pressure, enhances circulation and contributes to a healthier heart. It can help you lose weight by boosting your metabolism and helping you burn more calories even when you're not working out.

Most importantly, it'll make you feel like a *badass.*

How do I get started?

There are so many different ways to add weight to your workout – dumbbells, kettlebells and resistance bands, as well as specific machines in the gym. But you can get started without using any props, as the only weight you need is the weight of your own body. Starting this way is accessible, functional and convenient – you can do these moves from anywhere (and I mean literally anywhere). I promise you, body-weight exercises can really pack a punch. I still find many super challenging; it's a great way to test yourself and start building strength.

Your 15-minute full-body strength workout . . . using just your body weight

Set a timer to do each exercise for 40 seconds. It doesn't matter how many repetitions you manage in that time, because as your strength builds, you will be able to do it faster and faster and do more and more reps.

If you want to build up and test your abilities, you can repeat each round twice so that your workout becomes 30 minutes long.

ROUND 1: Upper body and core

Plank hold. Get down onto your forearms and toes (or hands, for a higher plank, if you prefer). Your body should be in a straight line from your head to your heels. Engage your core and glutes, don't let your hips sink down. Hold for 40 seconds, or for as long as you can manage! (See page 25.)

Walk-outs. Stand tall, hinge at the hips, then walk your hands out away from your feet to a high-plank position. Hold briefly, don't rush the move, then walk your hands back towards your feet and stand up. You could add a jump at the top or a modified push-up at the bottom if you're craving more challenge.

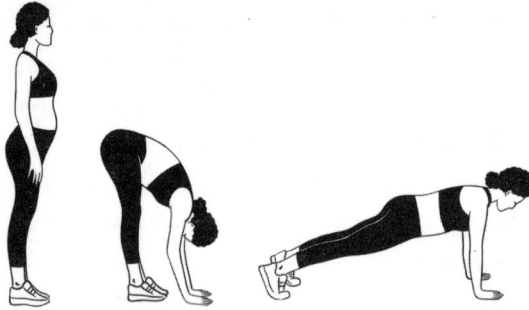

Modified push-ups with knees down. From a high-plank position (on your hands), drop your knees down to the floor. Keep a straight line from your head to your knees, then lower your chest to the floor with your elbows at a 45-degree angle. Engage your core and keep your hips level as you press back up.

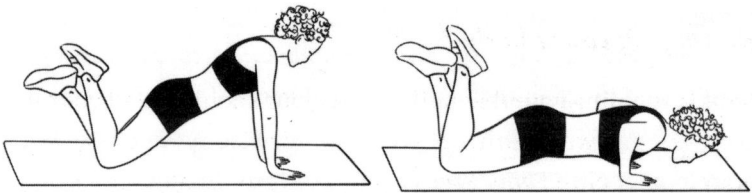

Shoulder taps. Back into that high plank, tap your right hand to your left shoulder, then place your hand on the floor again and tap your left hand to your right shoulder. Try to prevent your hips swaying by keeping your core engaged.

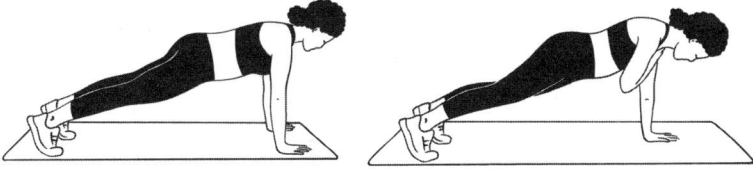

Superman hold. Lie down on your front with your arms extended out in front of you. Lift your arms, upper chest and legs off the ground to hold. Squeeze your glutes and back muscles – now hold for 40 seconds, and fly!

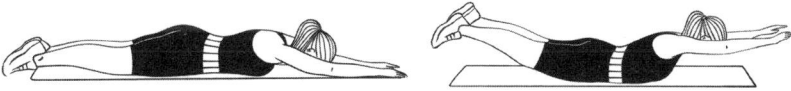

If you're going for the advanced option, repeat this round one more time.

ROUND 2: Lower body

Squats. Keeping your feet in line with your shoulders, sit your hips back as if you were sitting down in a chair. Keep your chest up and your knees behind your toes for proper form. Lift yourself back up with control. (See page 25.)

Reverse lunges (alternating). Step one foot back, then lower yourself down until both knees are at around 90 degrees. Push through the front heel to return to standing, then do the same on the other side.

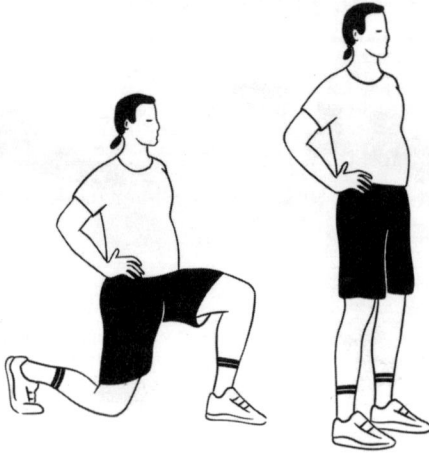

Wall sit. Lean back against a wall, then slide down it until your thighs are parallel to the floor. Your knees should be lined up above your ankles, with your back flat against the wall. Then hold for 40 seconds. This might sound easy, but it's really not!

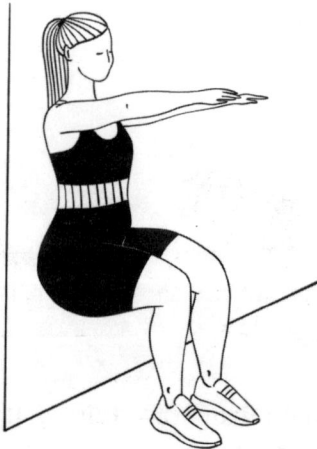

Calf raises. Stand up tall, raise your heels so that you are balancing on your toes, then lower slowly. Pause at the top for increased burn. This is another one that might seem easy, but it really tests both your strength and balance! (See page 23.)

Glute bridges. Lie on your back with your knees bent and your feet flat on the floor. Lift your hips by squeezing your glutes, then lower yourself back down again. Keep your shoulders connected to the floor and try not to arch your lower back.

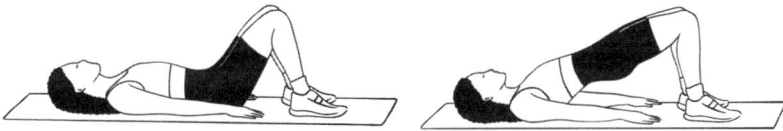

If you're going for the advanced option, repeat this round one more time.

ROUND 3: Core and conditioning to finish

Mountain climbers. From a high-plank position, drive your knees quickly towards your chest one at a time, back and forth. Keep your hips low and move fast. It's a little cardio boost to fire up your session.

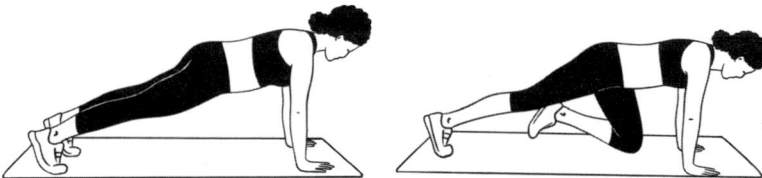

Lying leg raises. Lie on your back, raising alternating legs into the air and lowering them slowly without arching your back. To progress the move, try lifting both legs at the same time. And to improve your alignment and increase the intensity in your abs, put your hands under your hips.

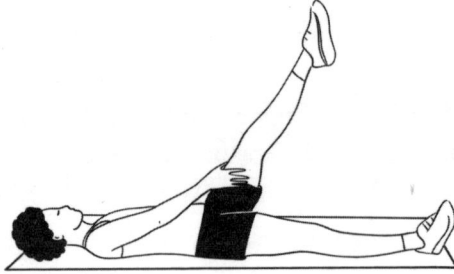

Side plank. To get into a side plank, start by lying on your side with your legs extended and stacked one on top of the other, with your feet flexed. Place your elbow directly under your shoulder, with your forearm flat on the floor at a 90-degree angle. Engage your core and lift your hips off the floor. If you're struggling, you could rest the top foot on the floor. Hold for 20 seconds. To take it one step further, add in a 'reach under' movement, where you reach your top arm under your body, then return it to your side. Repeat on the other side.

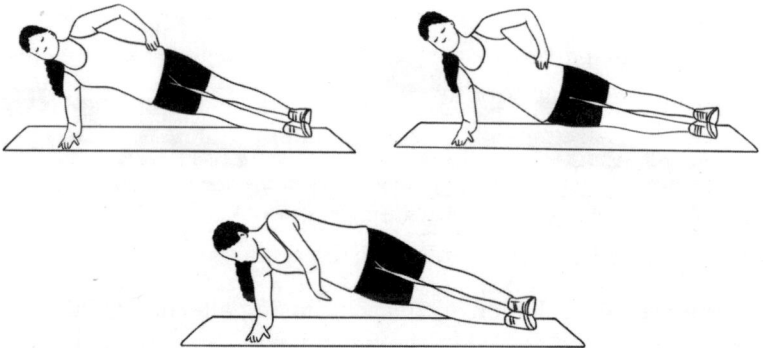

Dead bug. Lie on your back with your arms raised straight up above your shoulders and your knees at 90 degrees. Extend one leg, extend the opposite arm back behind your head, then return arm and leg to the starting position and switch sides. Ensure your lower back stays pressed into the floor.

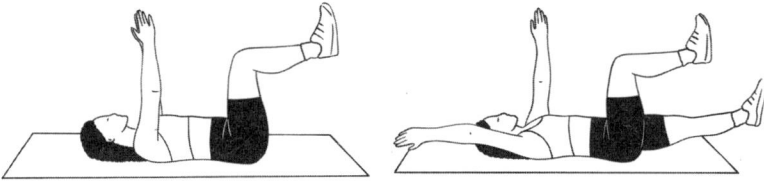

Squat with pulses. Perform a regular squat and then pulse gently, moving up and down three times before returning to standing.

If you're going for the advanced option, repeat this round one more time.

FUN: THE WINE BOTTLE WORKOUT

Now you've mastered strength-training using only your body weight, it's time to up the ante. And no, I'm not talking about using dumbbells. I'm talking about using wine bottles!

Just take a leaf out of my ol' mother's book – she loves wine, and she loves working those biceps, so why not combine the two? All you need for this workout is two bottles of vino and a sense of humour.

SAFETY WARNINGS: If you tend to get sweaty hands, I'd recommend wearing some kind of grippy gloves. Do this outside if you can in case of any spillage, and choose cheap bottles rather than your best sauvignon. Use red wine at your own risk!

Standing up with a wine bottle in each hand, complete 7 reps of each move below . . .

Bicep curl. Stand tall with your arms by your sides, holding both wine bottles. Curl them up to shoulder height, keeping your elbows close to your torso. Lower down with control.

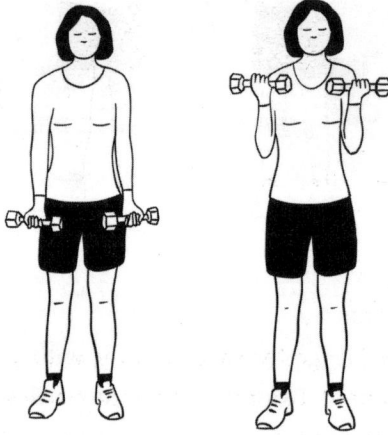

Half bicep curl. With your arms in the same starting position, lift up halfway so there's a 90-degree bend at the elbow and your forearms are parallel with the ground. Then lower down with control.

Top bicep curl. Now hold your arms at that halfway position and lift the wine bottles up to your shoulders, before lowering them back down to halfway.

Overhead shoulder press. Start with your elbows bent and your wine bottles at shoulder height. Lift your arms overhead until they are fully straight, then lower back down with control.

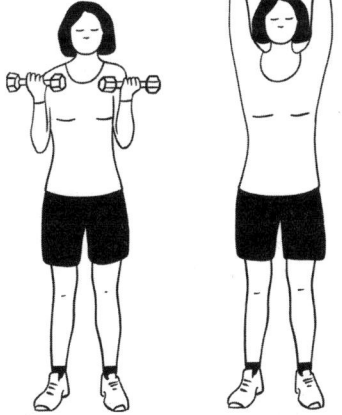

Tricep kickbacks. Hinge forward slightly, with your elbows tight to your sides and bent. Extend those wine bottles straight behind you, squeezing your triceps at the top. Slowly return to the bent position.

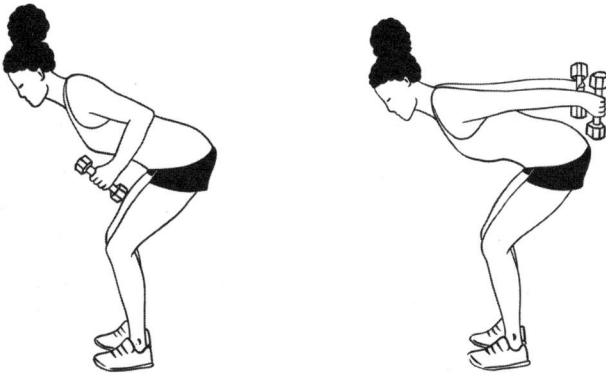

BONUS CHALLENGE:

Once you're done with the wine bottles, crack open one of them and fill up two glasses to the brim. Now repeat all the exercises holding a glass in each hand, trying your best to avoid spillage. (99 per cent of people will spill the wine doing this. But could YOU be that 1 per cent?!)

And finally . . . *drink the wine*. You've earned it.

NOURISH YOURSELF

FOCUS: MAKE FOOD A PRIORITY

By now, you've got some important focus points in check. Positive mindset? Check! Solid routine? Check! Now, I want to talk about something that you can do outside of your workouts that will ultimately support them and help them work a bit harder. No, I'm not talking about building an AI robot that can do your workouts for you – it's not that complicated, darling – I'm talking about the food you eat.

Before we go any further, let me make something clear: this is not a diet book, and I am not a nutritionist or a dietician. However, it goes without saying that movement isn't the only thing you can do to ensure a healthy body and mind. Supporting your body with nutritious and delicious foods wherever possible will also make a huge difference. If you want to tone up, build muscle, lose weight or you're just exercising for the mental health benefits, food can help with all of these things, too. Food and exercise are like sidekicks; they're the best of friends.

Food matters because, when you really boil it down, it's our fuel. But not all fuel is created equal. Some fuel has the power to fire us up and make us feel energised, while other fuel can slow us down and make us feel sluggish and unmotivated. In the same way you wouldn't put the wrong petrol into a shiny fast car, we should aim to fill our tanks with the *right* kinds of food. If we want to perform at our best, we need to have a look at the fuel we're guzzling. Is it helping us, or is it slowing us down and maybe leaking out all over the pavement? (Sorry, I may have taken the car analogy too far.)

I learned about the importance of food as fuel in my athlete days. Old Tommy Trotter would eat all sorts of sugary cereals and snacks before school, but while rugby training I learned to eat more carbs and protein as this would enhance my performance, making me stronger on the field. Although I don't necessarily eat like a rugby player anymore, I think about my food in a similar way: I want to give my body the nutrients it needs to stay well-oiled and functioning as it should.

They say 'you are what you eat', but I'm not convinced that's true – I am a human, not a chicken breast, thanks very much. But you definitely do *feel* what you eat. Everything you put in your body affects you in some way. It has some kind of impact on you – whether it's positive or negative. Sometimes, it can even be a mixture of both, and that's where my emphasis on balance comes in again. What really matters is that you shift your mind-set towards food, so you are viewing it as an essential fuel to support your health journey. It's not something to be afraid of or restrict. Food is an exciting, achievable and downright delicious piece of your fitness puzzle, and I'll show you how to get the best out of it.

The problem with diets

Unless you were born after the year 2000, you probably grew up being aware of (or being told to try) some kind of restrictive diet. There was the cabbage soup diet, which says you have to eat nothing but cabbage soup. And the banana diet, which suggested that you must eat nothing but bananas. And then there was the raw food diet, which says you shouldn't cook anything and only eat raw fruit and veg like a rabbit.

Even the less-bonkers diets would usually involve some element of calorie counting, 'don't eat this', and 'eat lots of this'. I'm not saying *all* diets are terrible – some do have scientific backing – but in general, most of the science these days shows that cutting out entire food groups and eating a lot of just one thing is not the way to go. In reality, eating a healthy diet is way more simple than we have been led to believe. It's about getting *more* of the good stuff onto our plates, into our mouths and into our bodies to fuel all our bodily processes.

First of all, I want you to repeat this after me: food is your friend, not your enemy. All those years of diet culture also taught us that we shouldn't eat 'too much'. In my opinion, it's not about eating 'too little' or 'too much', it's about quality, not quantity. *It's about giving your body what it needs to thrive.*

When I was in my unhealthy phase of chasing aesthetics in exercise, I was in a calorie deficit. This means I was burning more calories through exercise than I was eating. If you're overweight and trying to shed some pounds, it can be helpful to be in a calorie deficit. However, if the deficit is too extreme (which mine was), it can result in hormone imbalances, fatigue, muscle loss and even fertility issues. I had somehow forgotten that athlete's mindset of eating to fuel my performance, and I became a shell of my former self. It was only when I signed up for a marathon that I realised I *needed* that fuel, otherwise I physically wouldn't be able to race. That mindset shift was just what I needed – I started eating fuller, delicious portions, and started enjoying food again.

I can't even imagine slipping into those unhealthy habits again, because I remember just how drained and unhappy I was during that time. When you cut out food groups and restrict yourself, you reduce your energy and your potential. Not only that, but making drastic changes to your diet is difficult, unsustainable and much harder to stick to. Instead, I'm going to show you how you can tweak your diet to add more of what will make you feel good and support your workouts. We're not taking anything away altogether, we're only adding and modifying.

> NOTE: If you think that you, or someone you love, might be struggling with disordered eating (whether that's undereating, purging or binge-eating), it's okay not to be okay, and it's important to seek help. Either speak to your GP or contact a charity like Beat (beateatingdisorders.org.uk).

Here's what we're NOT gonna do . . .

Count calories. The recommended daily intake of calories is 2,500 per day for men, and 2,000 for women. That's the last thing I'm going to say about calories! It can be useful to have that overall number in your head, because if you know you're going all-out at dinner time, you can make healthier choices during the day. But you don't need to count every single calorie you eat – this is where obsession breeds, and obsession is unhealthy (take it from me!). And anyway, a healthy diet isn't always about calories – some things have higher calories but are rich in nutrients, healthy fats and protein. So don't get too hung up on the numbers.

Make dramatic changes. If you want to eat a vegan diet for ethical reasons, or cut out gluten because that's better for your gut, then more power to you! We all have our own dietary priorities and reasons. But generally speaking, in order to have a healthy diet, you don't *need* to cut out entire food groups to make changes. My approach is all about making easy and achievable tweaks to the diet you already have and the food you already love.

Here's what we *ARE* gonna do:

Make smarter choices. I'm going to give you lots of tips and suggestions throughout this chapter – but let's be honest, you already know most of this stuff. We've learned about eating healthy diets since we were little kids; we know that fresh ingredients are gonna be better for you than heading to the ready-meal section, digging out frozen chips or picking from the sweets and crisps aisle. If you're here, reading this book, you're already facing the reality of your choices so far, and you're willing to make different ones. Aye aye, captain!

Be conscious and mindful. Having a few crisps is totally fine. Opening a family bag of crisps and munching through the entire thing without even realising you've done it – not so fine. Mostly because you're doing this on autopilot, without even thinking. I genuinely respect you if you sit down and decide: 'Today, I am going to eat this entire bag of crisps, because I want to, and I deserve it.' Because at least you have thought it through and made a decision, rather than just eating something because it's in front of you. Eating well is just about consciously *noticing* what you're eating, knowing when to start and knowing when to stop. It's about being mindful about what we're eating and, importantly, *why* we're eating (for example, do you need nourishment and energy, or are you just bored?).

Enjoy food. Even though I have said that food is fuel, this isn't the only purpose it serves. Food also brings people together. It's communal, it's fun, it's the ultimate mood-booster. One thing you will not be hearing me say is, 'Skip that dinner with your friends so you can eat that boring meal prep in your freezer.' No, sir! Not on my watch! You should still enjoy food and the ceremony of eating. I don't want you to ever sacrifice that side of things. The trick is just to follow the two points above (making smarter choices and remaining mindful) so that you can keep your diet balanced. If you know you're getting a Chinese takeaway with your family for dinner, perhaps you'll make an extra effort to eat bowls of rainbow goodness for breakfast and lunch. You don't need to sacrifice that takeaway. Enjoy the hell out of it.

TROTTER TASK: KEEP A FOOD DIARY

Generally, I wouldn't recommend tracking your food too carefully because this can lead to obsession. However, as you set off on this journey I think it's useful to see where you're at. What are you currently eating? What are your habits? Keep a food diary for just one week, as a way to guide your healthier choices.

Write down (either on paper, or a note on your phone) what you're eating for breakfast, lunch and dinner – plus snacks – on each day of the week. If you can, include water, caffeine and drinks too (alcoholic and non-alcoholic).

I also want you to note down how you feel each day. Do you have an energy dip after lunch? Are you exhausted by 5 p.m.? Are you wired at bedtime?

Once you can see your diary, you can identify patterns and work out some easy ways to make changes.

- Do you buy processed snacks on the go?

- Is your breakfast sugary? Are you even having a proper breakfast?!

- Are you reaching for takeaways frequently because you're too busy to cook?

- Are you eating sweet snacks in the evenings before bed?

You don't need to know *what* to do with this information just yet – the next few pages will help you make adjustments. For now, you're armed with knowledge about your diet, which is the first step to making progress.

The truth about healthy food

If you want to get really technical about it, there are loads of different food groups, and each has their own unique benefits. But I'm a simple guy, so I like to keep things simple. The way I see it, good food can be divided into three categories: PROTEIN, CARBS and COLOUR. If your meals tick off each one, you know you're on the right track for a balanced, healthy diet.

PROTEIN

Our bodies need proteins. Why? Because they're the building blocks of all our organs, cells and tissues. So, it goes without saying that if we want healthy muscles and healthy bones, feeding our bodies with protein is the way to go. Not only that, protein releases energy gradually, meaning we stay fuller (and feel more revved-up) for longer. And another bonus? Some of the amino acids found in protein (like tryptophan) are needed to make neurotransmitters in the brain like serotonin (known as the body's 'happy' chemical). So protein can even enhance your mood.

So, what counts as protein?

There are loads of protein sources you can access by eating nutritious whole foods and without the need for powders or supplements! If you eat meat, the best kinds to include in your meals are *lean* meats – meaning cuts with minimal fat content, and which aren't processed with other ingredients (examples of processed meats are things like sausages and bacon). This is because they contain additional ingredients that perhaps aren't as good for you – such as extra gluten, fats and salt. Sticking to the lean stuff – like chicken and fish – where possible, just means you know exactly what you're absorbing, and you'll get a good amount of protein, vitamins and minerals without eating too much fat. Beans, pulses, grains, nuts and seeds (peanuts are a great source of protein), tofu and lots of veggies (such as broccoli and edamame) are also packed with protein!

And how much protein should I eat?

It's recommended that men eat 55g of protein per day and women eat 45g, but nobody has time to measure that, so I aim for a portion of protein in every meal. For breakfast, that could mean two scrambled eggs, or it might mean a bowl of yogurt with some extra peanut butter for good measure. At lunch, maybe that's a chicken breast in a salad, and at dinner a bean Bolognese. You don't need to go overboard, but when I'm training, I might add in some extra protein as snacks to keep me going. My idea of a protein snack would be apples dipped in peanut butter, or some cold chicken, as opposed to protein bars or shakes. Again, these are ultra-processed using a whole load of extra ingredients. Not necessarily *bad*, especially if you only have them now and again, but I always try to keep it simple where possible.

MY FAVOURITE PROTEIN SOURCES

Eggs

Natural yogurt

Cashew butter (in fact, any nut butter)

Oat milk (it contains less protein than cow's milk, but it is still a great source!)

Tins of kidney beans (and even baked beans)

Salmon fillets

Hummus and falafel (chickpeas are rich in protein)

Tofu

Roasted peanuts (for snacking)

Chicken

Steak

CARBS

If you grew up before the 2000s, you may have been led to believe that carbs = bad. I'm not exactly sure why these brilliant foods were demonised for so long, but it's time we put that right! Carbohydrates essentially provide your body with energy. When you're exercising, your body relies on this energy source even more.

What are carbohydrates?

Technically, a carbohydrate is a type of sugar molecule that is found in lots of different foods. But 'carbohydrates' as we know them describes a food group that contains particularly high-carb foods. They are also rich in fibre, which is important for healthy digestion. This food group includes rice and different types of grains, breads, pasta and starchy vegetables, including white and sweet potatoes.

Are all carbohydrates created equal?

Some types of carbs are considered superior when it comes to energy release and other beneficial nutrients. These are called 'complex carbohydrates', which means they are made up of long chains of sugar molecules and therefore release energy slowly and gradually, which is better for your body. Complex carbs include whole grains, potatoes (white and sweet) and legumes like lentils and chickpeas (notice how these are great sources of protein too? Double win!). By contrast, simple carbohydrates are digested and processed quickly by the body, which means you could feel hungry or sluggish again more quickly. Simple carbs generally include more processed foods, like white bread, cakes and pasta. This doesn't mean you should avoid these types of carbs, it just helps to be mindful. And, if you can, switching to brown rice, brown pasta and wholemeal bread can be an easy win. Or pair your simple carbs with good proteins and good colour to balance the books – for example, add chicken, tofu or salmon to your pasta dish plus plenty of veggies. That's how champions are made.

How many carbs should I eat per day?

Research suggests you need about 30g of carbohydrates each day to meet your energy needs. But the real-life quantities depend on the type of carb and what your objectives are. As a general goal, you could aim to have simple carbs in one meal each day (for example, a sandwich or a bowl of pasta), then choose complex carbs for your other meals (grains and sweet potatoes).

MY FAVOURITE CARBOHYDRATES

- Granola and oats for brekkie
- Brown seeded toast (to have with scrambled eggs in the morning)

- Roasted sweet potatoes
- Jacket potato
- Packets of microwaveable rice (for easy lunches)
- Brown pasta

COLOUR

This category catches all the essential vitamins and minerals we need to stay healthy, and to support our bones, organs, heart and mood. And they're pretty easy to spot: these are foods that come in every colour of the rainbow, and you find them in the fresh food aisle. I'm talking fruit and vegetables. Of course, everything in moderation, but generally speaking you can't get enough of these bad boys. The NHS recommends eating 5 portions of fruit and veg a day, but I say get in as many as you possibly can. Go bananas! (Literally.)

But also, try as much as you can to eat a good *selection* of fruit and veg. Research shows that your gut loves variety, so this is great if you have any digestive issues. Plus, different fruit and veg contain different quantities of essential vitamins and minerals. For example, citrus fruits are rich in immune-boosting vitamin C, dark leafy greens are high in calming magnesium, and berries are rich in antioxidants which help your body clean out toxins. So the more you can tick off, the more you're supporting your body with everything it needs.

MY FAVOURITE COLOURFUL FOODS

- Avocado (also a great source of healthy fat)
- Bananas (great on-the-go snacks)
- Carrots (both raw and cooked)
- Berries (great for adding to breakfast granola)
- Asparagus (but be warned about smelly wee)

- Grapes (and raisins – great for snacking)
- Leafy greens (kale and spinach are the GOATs)
- Pomegranate seeds (sprinkle on top of salads – et voilà!)
- Onion and garlic (always, for everything)
- Broccoli and cauliflower (these are great for your gut)
- Herbs and spices – basil, parsley, paprika, cumin, turmeric . . . the list goes on

If you're ticking off some good proteins, carbs and colour every day, you're onto a winner. However, there is just one more group that I want you to be aware of – I call this category TREATS.

TREATS

These are foods that are oh-so-delicious but contain ingredients that aren't always so great for your body and mind. This includes . . .

- Those simple carbs we talked about – white bread and pasta.
- Cheese – a good source of calcium and protein in moderation, but also high in fat and calories.
- Sugary foods, since sugar causes energy crashes (sweets, chocolate, cakes).
- Salty foods, as salt increases blood pressure (think crisps, pretzels, fast food).
- Saturated fats (these can lead to heart disease in big quantities) – including butter, palm oil and deep-fried foods that you might find in your favourite junk-food chain restaurants.
- Anything that is highly processed – those items that contain multiple ingredients and you don't even know what each of them are.
- Caffeine (having more than 2 cups of coffee or caffeinated drinks a day), as this has a lot of negative side effects,

including increased anxiety, digestive problems and increased blood pressure.

- Alcohol, since it damages your liver and increases risk of cancers (plus it often contains a lot of sugar).

These are not 'bad' foods and drinks. In fact, they're pretty *friggin' delicious* food and drink. Us humans are hard-wired to crave sugary, fatty and salty foods (and get pissed on wine) because it feels good in the moment. But the trick is to indulge in *moderation*. View them as treats and you won't reach for them every single day. And, to be honest, this will actually help you enjoy them even more. If you had the same thing every day, it would get boring, wouldn't it? Limit that fast-food takeaway to once a fortnight. Only drink booze on the weekends. Keep your coffee to the morning. Buy that frappuccino chai matcha latte with vanilla syrup, but maybe just once a month. Not only will they feel more special, it'll be better for your body, too.

NOTE: If you find you're treating yourself far too often, ask yourself the question: do I need this edible treat, or could I find some comfort in another way? Often, we reach for chocolate or ice cream out of habit, because it provides a safe space for us when we're feeling a certain way. If you can get to the bottom of *why* you reach for those treats all the time, and maybe replace them with something different (a phone call with a friend, or even a bowl of fruit instead), you might find yourself breaking the habit.

Get excited about food

Jeepers creepers, good food doesn't need to be boring. It's not like you need to live for the treats and just eat dull bowls of plain old rice and grilled chicken the rest of the time. That is simply no fun at all, and I won't allow it. The trick is to find easy, manageable meals that are good for you – and that you *actually really enjoy eating.* It might take a bit of trial and error, but I know you'll get there. Especially if you follow my top tips . . .

Experiment with recipes. View your evening cooking as an opportunity for an adventure. It's so easy to find healthy recipes these days – just go on TikTok and you'll find exactly what you're craving. Not only can this be fun (especially if you get a friend or partner involved), it can also help you fine-tune a collection of go-to recipes that you know are easy wins.

Have an open mind. One of my clients, Paula*, told me that she struggled to eat healthily because she was a fussy eater. She didn't like most fruit and vegetables. So I set her a challenge: each week, try a completely new fruit or vegetable she hadn't eaten much. She started with kale, then red cabbage, then kiwis. It turned out she didn't dislike fruit and veg, she was just a fussy kid and she didn't like *the idea of* fruit and veg. As she became more confident, she started reintroducing fruit and veg that she had absolutely decided she hated – including bananas and mushrooms. It turned out, she really didn't hate those either. A lot of the time, we tell ourselves we don't like things, and we can actually train ourselves to like things more. Our tastes change all the time – you just have to keep trying different foods. You never know, you might surprise yourself by how diverse your taste buds actually are.

Simplify your meal prep. Social media is full of people who spend their Sundays prepping every single meal for the week ahead. Sounds great, except then you've lost your Sunday Funday. Personally, I'd rather go for a run and hang out with my mates all day before the start of the week. If you're short on time on weeknights, what you *can* do is prep just one element: for example, popping a few seasoned breasts of chicken into the air fryer, or roasting some sweet potatoes. That way, you have *something* that you can easily add into your lunches (or dinners) as the week goes on. Go for easy wins like pre-packaged salads, microwaveable bags of grains and rice and pre-chopped fruit and veg. Chuck it all together and you have meal prep . . . but without actually having to do all of that prep. Result.

If it ain't broke . . . It's totally fine to stick to the same kinds of meals day-in, day-out. To be honest, I usually have the same breakfast on most days: scrambled eggs, with some granola, yogurt and fruit on the side. It's delicious, fills me up, and it ticks off my protein, carbs and colour. If it helps you to take the decision-making out of the process and have the same lunch every day in the office, you do that. You can also switch up your 'go-tos' in small ways – for example, swapping chicken for salmon, or rotating different vegetables. It's okay to find a structure that works for you and keep to it.

Easy hacks to level up your diet

I told ya that you don't need to make huge changes to make your diet healthier. And I meant it. Here are some easy ways to do it . . .

Cut caffeine. Have one cup in the morning, then switch your afternoon cup for decaf or a herbal tea.

Swap your oil. Instead of using vegetable oil, use olive oil. Also, go for a spray rather than a liquid. Using an air fryer is also a great way to save on added oil if you're frying or roasting.

Focus on breakfast. It really does set the tone for the rest of the day. A healthier breakfast – containing protein – means you're less likely to snack and crave treats for lunch. Start as you mean to go on!

Drink loads of water. Flush out those toxins and keep your energy levels stable with good old-fashioned H_2O. Aim for 6–8 glasses per day. If you find water boring, try adding fruit or cucumber for a flavoured kick.

Don't add sugar to your tea, coffee or matcha. Instead, try a sweeter milk – for example, oat milk – if you need that sweet fix.

Don't add salt to your meals once they're on your plate. Add salt when you're cooking (seasoning is important, guys, I'm not an animal), but you don't need to overdo it.

Add an extra portion. If you're feeling particularly hungry, on workout days, or maybe before your period if you're someone who has those, allow yourself a little more food. 'Going up for seconds' might be viewed negatively, but it's actually better to fill up on those healthy proteins, carbs and colours than add in extra treats just because you're hungry.

DO YOU NEED TO TAKE SUPPLEMENTS?

There are tons of pills, powders and potions on the market that claim to make you fitter and healthier, but what do you *actually* need?

Personally, I prefer to get most of my protein, vitamins and minerals from the food I eat, rather than using concoctions that are filled with all kinds of ingredients that I can't even read the names of.

That said, you might want to top up specific vitamins and minerals, as some aren't always so easy to get from your diet alone. For example, the NHS recommends supplementing vitamin D, which is so important for your bones and energy levels (especially during winter, but it's useful all year round if you live somewhere with low sunlight levels, like Blighty, or your work hours mean you don't get outside enough).

If you're vegan, you may need to take a B12 supplement (again, so important for energy), since this can only be found in animal products. Many of us also don't eat enough probiotic foods, so taking an extra probiotic daily could work wonders for your gut.

Do your research based on your own health baselines, consult your doctor and find out which vitamins and minerals could be worth topping up. You don't need to take a supplement just because it's a trend.

FEAR: MAKE FRIENDS WITH FAILURE

We all have those moments we would describe as failures. Maybe you didn't land the promotion you wanted. Maybe you didn't manage to save your relationship. Maybe, like my mate, you failed your practical driving test several times in a row.

These feelings of 'failure' – of not getting the thing you wanted – can really sting. It's not a nice feeling, is it? Even thinking about occasions that happened long, long ago can trigger those raw feelings again – maybe of embarrassment, or self-doubt.

It's understandable that you might want to avoid ever feeling like a failure again. So what do you do? You stay well away from any possibility of failure. You stick to what is 'safe'. Because you think that if you can't achieve exactly what you want, and do it perfectly, it's better not to bother trying at all. And if we *do* try and then fail, we very quickly retreat and give up. When we fear failure, we become stranded and frozen.

This is a common underlying fear with so many of my clients. When they say they're afraid of exercising, what they're really saying is that, underneath it all, they're afraid of failing. They're scared of showing up and trying, and having nothing to show for it. They're scared of being the slowest or the weakest. They're scared of what others will think of them. All of this leads back to a fear of failing.

But with my approach it isn't possible to fail; it's only possible to learn. You see, 'failure' implies it's the end of the story. If you were watching a film and the heroes failed their mission midway through, but then ended the film triumphant, did they really fail? No! They used that 'failure' as a tool to learn. That tool ultimately leads towards their victory. It was actually an *essential stepping stone* towards the film's happy ending.

The way I see it, if you keep going after a failure, it's not a failure – it's just a setback. And guess what? Setbacks are necessary. They help us recalibrate. They help us reassess. They give us motivation to move forward. With my plan, you simply *can't* lose – you either win, or you keep going. It ain't over til it's over, baby!

With this in mind, I want to show you how you can reframe failures as steps along your journey. I want you to see them as something to embrace, to welcome and to learn from. It's time to kick that fear up the backside and send it into outer space.

Create the opportunity for success

I don't think you should avoid failure. I say, run at it – head on! Charge that unicorn! However, I do think that sometimes we set ourselves up for failures that simply aren't necessary. And it's all down to how we frame what a 'success' and what a 'failure' look like.

First of all, we tend to measure what is 'successful' by someone else's yardstick. I know that I have been guilty of this. I have set myself goals for marathons with extremely fast times because I have seen someone else do it (there's that super-competitive, dog-with-a-bone Tommy again!). But success looks different for everyone. I have since realised that completing a marathon *regardless of the time* is a bloody huge success in itself. Even if it takes 10 hours, that's still a success, because you have beaten all of the other people who never tried to begin with.

Then there's the fact that we set ourselves time-restricted targets and goals that are numbers-based. Maybe you want to lose X amount of weight by a certain month. Or maybe you want to run a 5k in less than 25 minutes. I'm all for setting these goals – it's good to have something to work towards – but it's also very important to be realistic with yourself. Where are you starting from? What's the likelihood that you can actually achieve this? Are you setting yourself up for failure by trying to pursue such a restrictive goal that you're bound to disappoint yourself?

I see this all the time with my clients. One such client was George*. He had a habit of starting new exercise regimes in January, then quitting them by the end of February. It wasn't that he was incapable of sticking to an exercise routine, it's just that he lacked patience. He wanted to see results by the end of February, and when he didn't, he became frustrated and had no motivation – so he gave up. When he started with me, I told him: 'If you never stop, you'll never fail.' Once we peeled back that restrictive idea of 'seeing results by February', and kept the goal much more open-ended, George was able to get into a steady rhythm. And guess what? By the summer, he had dropped a dress size. If you're not seeing results right now, it doesn't mean you're failing, it just means you're still on your way.

Keep your goals fluid and ongoing, rather than restrictive, then the only option is to succeed.

You don't always get what you want – but you get what you need

A few years ago, I signed up for a half marathon. As someone who had done a lot of races by that point, I was pretty confident in how it would go. I would fly like the wind! But on this occasion, it didn't quite work out like that.

At some point during the race, my knee gave out. Normally I could just shake this out and keep powering on, but for some reason my body said: *Nope.* So I walked/limped the rest of the way to the finish line. At first, my brain told me that I had failed. I was aiming for a certain time, I wanted to beat my personal best, and I ended up with the slowest time I could've imagined.

But I quickly realised that this wasn't a failure – it just wasn't what I needed at that time. Instead, that race taught me a different, valuable lesson. It taught me the importance of patience, of slowing down, and of listening to my body. For years, I had pushed through pain, but this was the first time I didn't have a choice. Limping to the finish line was actually strangely powerful; I felt empowered by my own resilience. Now, I see that it was a blessing that I 'failed' that day.

I'm sure you can look back at some of the biggest failures in your life and think: *Wow, that was a blessing in disguise!* Maybe you didn't get a job you desperately wanted, but then another, even better one came along. Or maybe you had your heart broken by the person you thought was the one, only to meet the *actual* love of your life and realise that they really weren't. It's difficult to know what's coming next when we're in the moment, when we feel that hit of pain or sadness from failing. But when you look back, you generally view those failures as blessings.

Keep this in mind the next time you feel like you've hit the floor. *I wonder how this blessing is going to reveal itself? I wonder WHEN it will reveal itself? Maybe next month. Maybe next year. I will look back on this moment and be glad it happened.* Even if you don't believe it right now, tell it to yourself anyway.

Failures = lessons

I've already spoken a bit about how you can *learn* from your failures to come back stronger. And if you really want to dig into that, we could just do away with the word failure altogether and replace it with the word 'lesson'. Yes, that's right. Put the word 'failure' in the bin.

If we view failures as lessons, we use them as moments to take a look at our growth, rediscover our motivation and remind ourselves that we can do hard sh*t. Lessons aren't always easy, but blimmin 'eck, they are valuable. I bloody hated most of my lessons at school, but thank God I learned to read and write, because here I am, writing this book for you! Lessons are hard, but they make us well-rounded people.

When my rugby career ended, that could've been considered a failure. It was something I had worked towards my whole life and I didn't get the chance to reach my pinnacle. But I look back on my rugby years as nothing but lessons; I learned how to be a team-mate, how to push myself to my limits, and it helped me to discover my life's purpose – to help people get fit. It was the best classroom to prepare me for this rollercoaster we call life.

Every time you have a moment that feels like failure, ask yourself: what is this setback teaching me? How can I use it to push me, and motivate me to do better?

Magnify the successes

We live in a world that celebrates successes and hides failures. You see the actor winning the Oscar, but you don't see how many failed auditions they went through before they got their big break. You see the bestselling book, but you don't see how many drafts and first attempts came before it (*trust me*). You see the hotshot CEO, but you don't see that they were an intern once, constantly getting things wrong.

The most successful and admirable people you know didn't have a smooth ride. Of course, privilege plays a role in success, and for some people success does just come extremely easy (lucky buggers). But for most people, there are a lot of failures behind every success. You just don't see all the times that person had to pick themselves up and try again. But trust me, they did.

From speaking to a lot of successful people, I have noticed that a big thing they have in common is *optimism*. They celebrate the successes more than they cry over the failures. Remember I said you should always try to do 1 per cent better than you did yesterday? This kind of mindset, where you're constantly growing and improving, will guard against the pain of setbacks. Because even if you fall back a bit, you're still on an upward curve. And that, my friend, is what counts.

TROTTER TASK: NOTE YOUR WINS AND WORK-ONS

Every time you go for a workout, jot down one win and one work-on:

Your win = Something that you achieved. For example, you shaved 30 seconds off your run time, you lifted a heavier weight, did an extra squat, feel more comfortable and at ease with your workouts. Even if you think you've had a 'bad' workout, you can train your brain towards thinking positively, because, guaranteed, there's definitely a win in there somewhere.

Your work-on = Something that you want to improve next time. It's not about berating yourself. It's not a failure; it's just something you want to get better at. Maybe you're still using a light resistance setting on an exercise bike and you want to increase it next time. Maybe you want to get through your reps faster or run a bit further.

When you look back over your notes, you might just find that your work-ons become wins in no time!

FITNESS: YOGA & PILATES

If you're already chomping at the bit to get started on some running or heavy cardio – love that for you, but let's slow down a little. I want to focus on an aspect of fitness that many of us overlook (particularly men), but that's so, so important for overall strength and longevity. These are the kinds of exercises that focus on building flexibility (the ability to stretch and lengthen your muscles) and mobility (the range of movement through your joints). Both of these together essentially make movement feel *easier, more comfortable and less restrictive*. Many workouts will include aspects of flexibility and mobility, but two of the best disciplines come in the form of low-intensity exercises like yoga and Pilates.

For some reason, yoga and Pilates are often seen as more 'feminine forms' of exercise. I know that, in the past, as a rugby bloke, I didn't think these kinds of exercise were *for* me. How wrong I was! Not only are these disciplines very welcoming to *everyone*, they're also mega beneficial. Recently, I've become a Pilates convert. Ever since my spinal injury (more on that in Level 4), I've learned just how important it is to focus on the inner, hidden muscles that you won't always reach in a standard strength-training sesh, but that you can activate during Pilates. Essentially, you build up your inner reserves, which can then support any other kind of exercise you do – from endurance running to lifting heavy weights.

The moves might look simple and slow from the outside – sometimes it's just a tiny curve in your spine or a slight pulse of your leg – but good golly, they can be brutal. I always thought my partner was off on a jolly when she went off to her Reformer Pilates classes with her iced matcha latte, but now I understand just how difficult, yet powerful, these kinds of moves are. I am not ashamed to say that I am humbled on the daily by Pilates.

What I love about yoga and Pilates is that you can easily get started from home. All you need is an exercise mat – you don't even need a pair of trainers, as you can usually be barefoot. So it's totally possible to get comfortable with the moves before attending a class, and you can do quick sessions that are as short as 10 minutes long that can still make such a huge difference to how limber and stable you feel over time.

If you're not familiar with either yoga or Pilates, allow me to explain what they are and how they can benefit you – and then I'll share some of the best moves to get started. Trust me, these disciplines will change the way you see exercise. They're mood-boosting and calming, yet challenging and exciting. The perfect combo, in my humble opinion.

YOGA

What is it? It's a mind-body practice with ancient roots that combines movement with breathing and awareness. It includes flowing through physical poses in combination with breathwork.

When you picture yoga, you might imagine people in fancy poses where they look like human pretzels, but the basis of yoga is really all about staying present through movement. There are lots of different types of yoga that serve different purposes. Hatha and yin yoga are mostly for stretching and relaxation, while vinyasa and dynamic yoga types involve moving through poses quickly, and you can actually work up a sweat. You can find many core yoga moves in other workouts – especially during warm-ups and cool-downs. Moves like cat cow, downward dog, forward folds and low-lunge stretches are all key parts of yoga. See? Not so intimidating.

What does it help with?

It's one of the best things you can do for flexibility – many yoga moves stretch out your muscles and improve your range of motion. If you struggle to do some of the moves at first because you feel inflexible, well, that's even more reason to do it!

You'll improve your strength using just your bodyweight – especially in your core, arms, legs and postural muscles. Even better, it helps to strengthen smaller stabilising muscles that often get overlooked in other workouts.

Many yoga moves (including tree pose and warrior variations) are fantastic for improving balance and coordination, which can help prevent falls and injury.

So much of yoga is about posture – even when you're sitting down and breathing quietly. And good posture can help you maintain good form in other disciplines of exercise.

Thanks to the fact that you link up movement with breath, it's a great form of stress relief. Lots of people say it brings them mental clarity and a sense of peace.

Slower forms of yoga can be seen as a form of moving recovery, allowing you to slow down and listen to your body.

PILATES

What is it? Pilates is a form of low-impact exercise that focuses on core strength, careful control and proper body alignment. It was developed by a guy called Joseph Pilates in the late 1920s as a method to help people build a strong and mobile body, with a specific emphasis on reducing injury. The movements are usually slow and controlled, and they can be done on a mat without any equipment, but they can also use props including a ring, a bouncy ball, resistance bands and, of course, the Reformer machine, which uses a carriage and differently-weighted springs to adjust intensity, add resistance and offer support. Pilates moves might seem simple but they're actually very detailed – you need to engage the right muscles during a given move, otherwise you may not notice the benefits. But if you get it right, it's amazing for your mind and body. Think of Pilates like installing the upgrade on your phone – except for your body. Everything will run more smoothly once you've done it.

What does it help with?
Pilates targets your deep, inner abdominal muscles – and a strong core helps with everything from weight-lifting to running.

Also focusing heavily on posture, Pilates can improve the way you stand, walk and sit, which results in less discomfort in your back and neck.

Focusing on inner muscles, Pilates improves stability and helps protect against injury. It's especially helpful for those with back pain or joint issues.

It strengthens your pelvic floor, which can improve the way your bowel and bladder function, plus it can even improve sexual function (oo-er).

As a low-impact form of exercise, it's great for gentle rebuilding – especially if you're coming off the back of injury or postpartum.

It balances your body, especially if your muscles are tight or overtrained.

YOUR 20-MINUTE YOGA–PILATES FUSION WORKOUT

This workout is the perfect way to stretch out your muscles and sync to the breath, while also packing a spicy punch.

ROUND 1: Yoga warm-up (5 minutes)

Cross-legged seated stretch. (1 minute) Sit cross-legged on the floor (or up on a cushion or block if your hips are tight). Sit tall through your spine to straighten your back. Inhale and reach your arms up over your head. Exhale, twisting to one side and dropping your hands down. Then inhale to go back up again, and exhale as you twist to the other side.

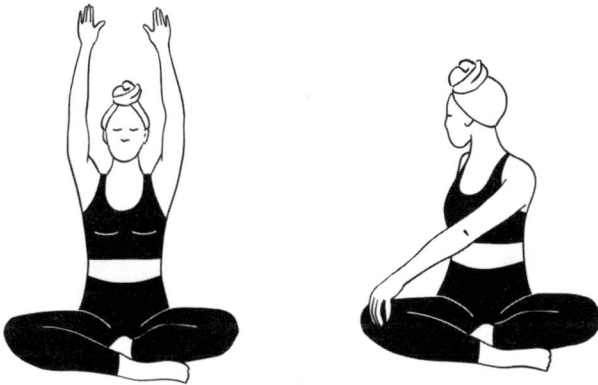

Cat-cow stretch. (1 minute) Come onto your hands and knees into tabletop position – shoulders in line with your wrists and hips in line with your knees. Inhale to drop your belly down, lift your chest and stick out your bum (Cow pose). Then exhale to round your spine into a curve, tucking in your chin (Cat pose).

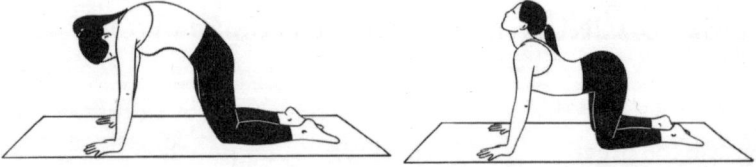

Forward fold into mountain pose. (1 minute) From standing, fold forward from the hips and reach down towards the ground – your hands don't need to touch the floor. Let your head hang loose, then roll up your spine slowly, one vertebra at a time, to standing. Stand tall in mountain pose, inhaling as you lift your arms into the sky, then exhale to slowly roll back down as you rolled up.

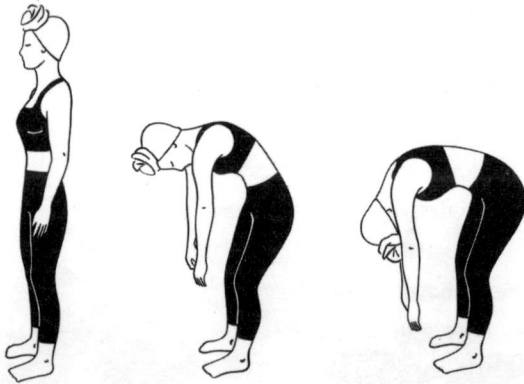

Downward dog. (1 minute) This is a classic yoga stretch that works the calves, hamstrings, spine and shoulders. From your hands and knees (tabletop position), tuck your toes under and lift your hips up and back. Your body should look a bit like an upside-down 'V'. Press your hands into the mat and your feet down towards the floor (it's okay if your heels don't touch the ground). Bend your knees one by one and wiggle back and forth to 'take your dog for a walk'. This stretch can feel tough at first, but it gets much easier with time.

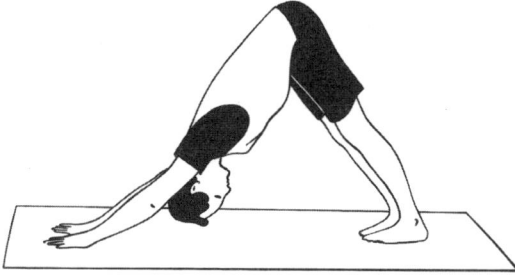

Low lunges. (30 seconds on each side) From downward dog, step your right foot forward between your hands and lower your back knee. Keep your front knee over your front ankle. Raise your arms up for a slight back bend. Switch sides after 30 seconds. To progress, try lifting the back knee so you're in a high lunge.

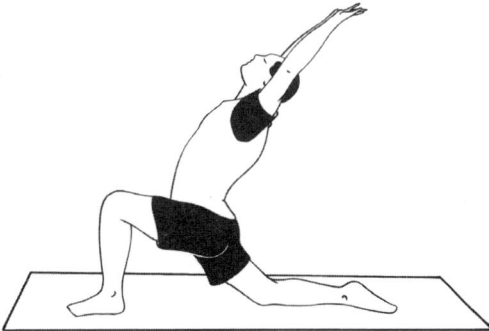

ROUND 2: Pilates core work (5 minutes)

Hundreds. (2 minutes) This classic Pilates dynamic warm-up is not for the faint-hearted. Lie on your back and lift your legs into tabletop (with your knees over your hips and shins parallel to the floor). Lift your head and shoulders off the mat, staying engaged in your core so you don't hurt your neck. Extend your arms by your side and pulse them up and down, with your palms facing towards the floor. Inhale for 5 pulses, exhale for 5 pulses, then repeat 10 times so you get to 100 pulses. If this is too intense, keep your head and shoulders on the floor, or lower your feet to the ground.

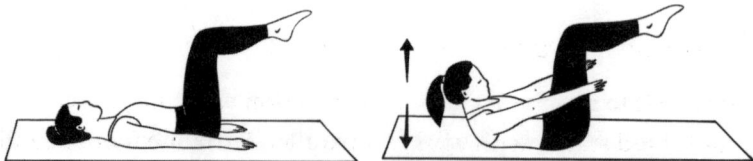

Single leg raises. (45 seconds on each side) Lie on your back with both legs straight. Bend one of your legs and place the foot on the floor for support, before lifting up the other leg in a straight line. Breathe as you lift it up and exhale as you lower it down with control, keeping your belly button pulled in towards the floor. Then swap sides.

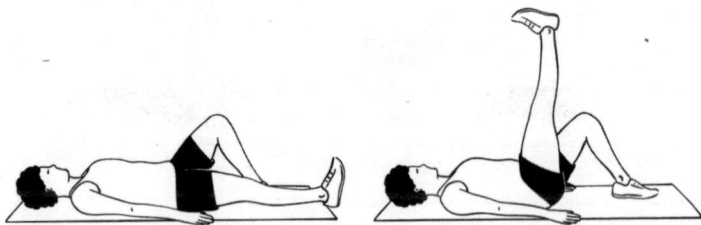

Clam legs. (45 minutes on each side) Lie on your side, with your knees bent, heels together and your hips stacked. If you're on a mat, your shins should be in line with the edge of it, at a 90-degree angle. Keeping your feet together, lift your top knee like a clam opening. Try not to let your hips roll back. Switch sides after 45 seconds (and slap your glute for a little shake-out if you need it).

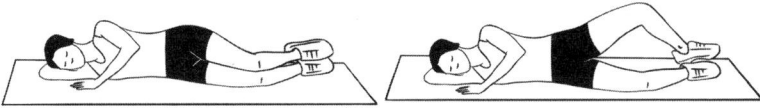

ROUND 3: Strengthening warrior flow (5 minutes)

Warrior II to reverse warrior. (2 minutes on each side) Stand in a wide-legged stance with your feet parallel. Turn one foot out and bend the knee to 90 degrees (this becomes your front foot). Keep your back leg straight and extend your arms out to the sides, looking over your front hand. This is warrior II. Hold here for 1 minute, then reverse your warrior by doing a windmill motion so that your back arm reaches down to touch your back leg and your front arm reaches up to the sky. Hold for 1 minute, then return to warrior II. Now switch sides and repeat on the other leg.

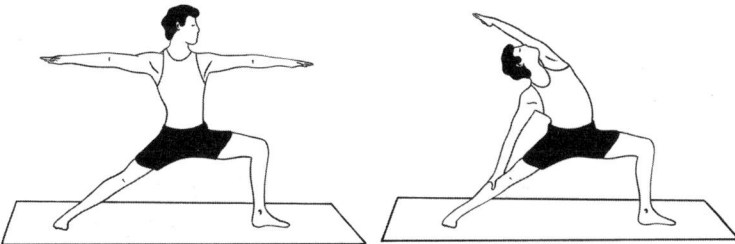

Chair pose to forward fold. (1 minute) From standing, with your feet together (or hip-width apart if that's more comfortable), bend your knees and sit your hips back just like you're sitting in a chair. Raise your arms overhead, hold for as long as you can, breathing deeply, then drop your head over your knees and release, bringing you back into a forward fold.

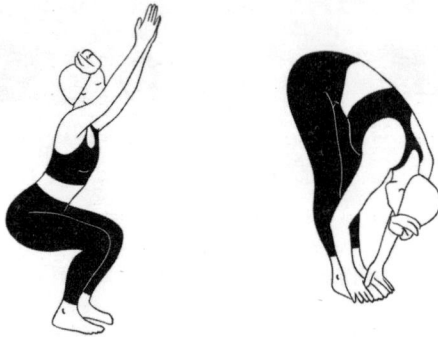

ROUND 4: Stretchy strong finisher (5 minutes)

Pigeon pose. (1 minute on each side) From tabletop position or downward dog, bring one knee forward towards the wrist on the same side and plant it down on the floor. Stretch the other leg back behind you. Stay upright or fold over your bent leg. This is an amazing deep stretch in the hips, glutes and lower back. After 1 minute, repeat on the other side.

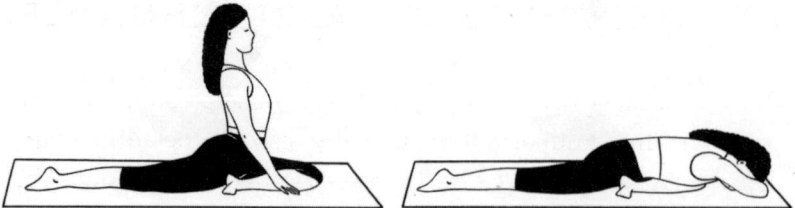

Glute bridge. (2 minutes) A classic move in both Pilates and yoga – great for strengthening your pelvic floor and core and reducing pain in the lower back. Lie on your back with your knees bent and your feet flat on the ground. Inhale to prepare, then exhale to press into your feet and lift your hips up. Squeeze at the top – you could even clasp your hands underneath you to deepen the stretch. Either stay there or gently lift and lower with control. (See page 49.)

Happy baby. (1 minute) Lie on your back, then bend your knees and bring them towards your chest. Grab the outsides of your feet with your hands, open your knees wide and flex your feet towards the sky, rocking from side to side. If that's too challenging, you can do the same thing but wrap your arms around your shins.

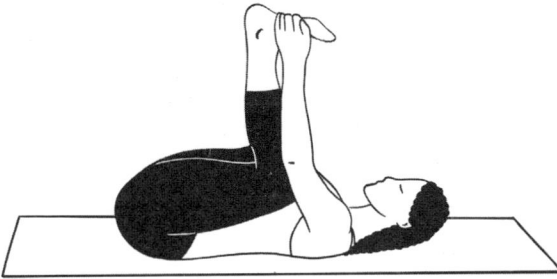

FUN: THE LOVE YOURSELF BALANCE CHALLENGE

One of the biggest perks of yoga is that it can help to improve your balance. This is important for so many reasons, including injury prevention, a stronger core and better coordination. So, this challenge is all about putting your balance to the test.

Remember we spoke about getting comfortable with failure, and viewing failures as lessons and stepping stones along your journey? Well, balance is a good way to put this training into action. When you start trying to balance, you're very likely to wobble and fall over the place. In fact, even the most experienced yogis will tell you that they embrace the wobbles. It's all a bit of fun and a good opportunity for humility.

So here's what we're gonna do. Below, I've listed instructions for five different balancing poses; starting with a beginner pose, then progressing to intermediate and advanced. You can stay on each pose for as long as you feel comfortable, practising as much as you like. You'll notice improvements really quickly if you spend five minutes on it every day! The trick is to focus on your breath, keep your eyes set on a fixed point in the distance (or the floor, depending on your pose) and let the wobbles come, but try your best to stay grounded through your standing leg.

But there's a twist! Rather than simply holding each pose for as long as you can muster, I want you to shout 'I LOVE MYSELF' from the top of your lungs, on repeat, each time you do it. Speaking (or shouting) challenges your balance even further, because it disrupts your breath control (which is a key way to stay upright), diverts your attention and activates the nervous system. It's *also* challenging because we rarely say that, don't we? But 'I LOVE MYSELF' is a powerful reminder to give yourself the credit for showing up, giving it a go and maintaining that self-acceptance, even when you fall.

Tree pose. Stand tall and shift your weight onto one foot. Lift the other foot so it's pressing against your ankle, calf or thigh (the higher you go, the harder it is, but just avoid the knee). It should look like a sideways triangle. Focus on a fixed point in front of you. Put your hands in prayer position at your heart, or lift them up into the air for a more advanced version. Swap over to the other side (you'll usually find that one side feels easier).

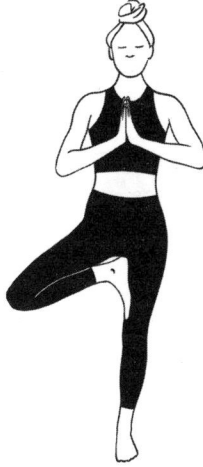

Heel-lifted chair pose. From standing with your feet together, sit your hips back into chair pose. Once you feel stable there, rise onto the balls of your feet and hold. Keep your knees together, with your arms straight, extended forward or overhead.

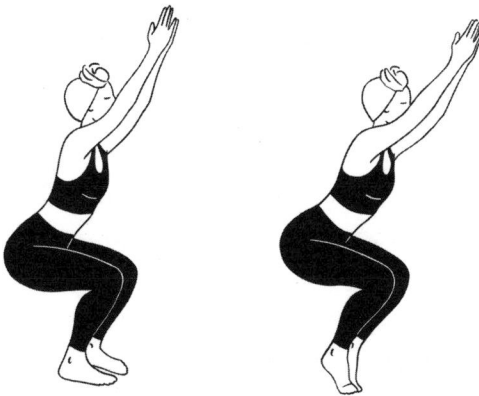

Warrior III. From standing, hinge forward from your hips while lifting one leg straight behind you. Look towards the ground, with your torso and back leg forming one long line. Have your hands in prayer position at your heart, or reach your arms to the side and back, like you're flying. Then switch sides.

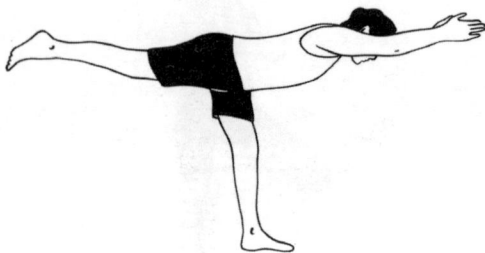

Half moon. Starting from warrior II, shift your weight onto your front foot and float your back leg up. With the arm that matches the side of your front foot, reach down towards the ground while the other arm lifts up to the sky. Open your chest sideways, stacking your hips and shoulders and looking up at your raised hand. Then switch sides.

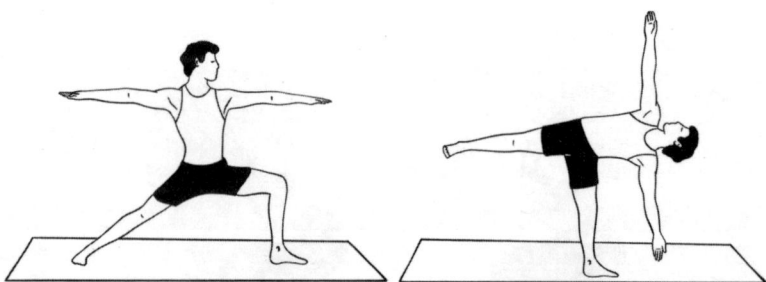

Standing hand-to-big-toe pose. Stand tall, then lift one leg and grab your big toe with your hand on the same side. Straighten that leg forward, or out to the side (but it's okay if it doesn't fully straighten). Engage your core and ground down into that standing leg. Repeat on the other side.

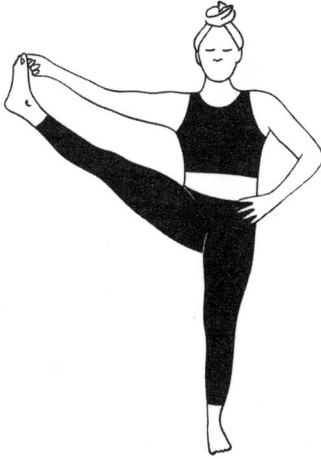

GO, GO, GO!

FOCUS: PRIORITISE VARIETY

They say that variety is the spice of life – and it couldn't be more true. Life is far more fun and exciting when we hang out with a variety of people, travel to different places and try new things.

But when it comes to exercise, many of us tend to get stuck in ruts. We choose the one type of exercise that we like (or believe we're capable of doing), then we stick to that. In the past, I have been guilty of that too. Especially if I'm training for a race, I'll get fixated on only running, cycling or whatever else it is that I'm trying to achieve. Dog. With. A. Bone.

I'm not saying there's anything wrong with that, in certain circumstances. It's an athlete's mentality, which I learned in my rugby days. Rugby training was highly specific, designed to enhance our performance on the field. Doing anything that deviated from that training plan could potentially reduce our athletic performance (and no one wanted that). But here's the thing: *if you're not an athlete, you don't need to train like one. You can train like a human.*

At the end of the day, most of my clients come to me because they want to feel better overall. They want to lose weight, improve their mental health and feel more content in their own skin. They aren't trying to meet one specific physical target, which means they shouldn't be only doing one specific physical activity. Some clients come to me because they *are* working out but they're not seeing the results they want. And often, it's because they're doing too much of one thing. They're too comfortable with what they know. They aren't willing to step outside their usual comfort zones.

I want to show you why this is so important. This Focus section is all about adding variety to your exercise routine. Spicing it up. Working across different disciplines. Trying new things as you go along. Adding new strings to your bow. Becoming a many-tricks unicorn.

In Level 2, you created space in your calendar to get in shape, but you may still be doing the same old moves every time. Now, I want to encourage you to get creative with that routine – ensuring it feels spicy, varied and keeps you interested. I can guarantee this will help create your healthiest body ever and allow you to get the most out of fitness. Bosh!

What is cross-training and why is it good for you?

Cross-training is basically a fancy way of saying 'doing different types of exercise'. It's considered the best way to improve your overall fitness, since different types of exercise have different benefits.

For example, you already know that strength-training is best for your bones and muscles, and yoga and Pilates are best for improving flexibility, mobility, balance and coordination. Hopefully, you also know that cardio exercises are best for increasing your overall fitness and burning calories. Not only that, but changing the *way* you exercise can have different benefits. For example, fast, short bursts are best for shedding pounds, while slow and steady workouts improve endurance and can lower your heart rate so that exercising feels less like hard work. Having a mix of *all* these different types of exercise in your routine, in some way or another, is a great way of ensuring you're hitting all these key markers of good health.

Plus, all the skills you gain in one aspect of fitness are transferable – meaning they'll help you in another aspect of fitness. If you have strong legs from strength-training and a strong core from Pilates, this will help your running technique. If you have strong arms from lifting weights, you might find it easier to attempt some powerful moves (like headstands) in yoga. Even a leisurely stroll through the park can help your more vigorous training as it can stabilise your heart rate. It's all beneficial. Nothing goes to waste. Move in all sorts of different ways and your body will love you for it.

A varied exercise routine also, importantly, protects against injury, because it ensures you never overtrain specific muscles and joints. We'll come back to this in the Fear section on page 102, which is all about preventing injury.

And finally, engaging in different types of training keeps things interesting. One of the main reasons my clients have given up in the past is quite simply that they get bored. They don't enjoy doing the same old moves in the same old gyms forever and ever. They ultimately want to challenge themselves, get creative and discover new sides to themselves that they didn't know existed. Although, much of the time they don't *know* that this is what they want.

Take, for example, my client, Penny*. In her mid-fifties, Penny wanted to lose some weight. She didn't understand why she had gained a few extra pounds, since she went on long, rambling walks and hikes almost every day with her two dogs. She told me she absolutely, hands-down, would *never* join a gym or go to an exercise class because she only liked to exercise outdoors. That said, she also refused to run because she had sore knees, and she didn't want to cycle because she was worried about safety and falling off her bike. She knew she probably needed to do some cardio exercise to meet her goals, but she'd put herself in a restrictive box that decided what she 'could' and 'couldn't' do.

After a lot of convincing, Penny finally agreed to attend a spinning class. This meant she could use a bike without worrying about being on the roads or falling off. Plus, I really hoped she might have fun with the choreography and loud music (she told me she often plugged into pop music on her long walks). I basically had to drag her into that class kicking and screaming, but guess what? She *loved* it, and she couldn't wait to go back. So that's exactly what she did – again and again. And once she felt more confident on her spin bike, she built up the courage to try a 'legs, bums and tums' class that focused on strength and toning. Before she knew it, she had a balanced routine made up of cardio and strength, and she still got to enjoy her daily walks. Finally, she achieved the results she wanted – and she gained so much more than that besides; an exercise routine she enjoyed, more strength to carry her new grandson and, better still, increased confidence in what she was *truly capable of.*

Penny is proof that you don't know what you don't know. As scary as it is to try something different, it's also full of promise, because you just never know what will set your heart alight and get you excited about fitness, possibly for the first time ever. No matter where you are in your fitness journey, it's *always* admirable to try something new. I already mentioned that I only recently added Pilates to my repertoire – and by golly do I respect those Pilates pros. Now, it's an important part of my routine.

Having an open mind with the exercise you do will only ever serve you well. It will reduce boredom, challenge your brain (which is especially important as you get older) and keep your body fighting-fit for longer. Tick, tick, tick! What's not to love?

The secret to a varied exercise routine

In Level 3, I told you that the secret to a balanced diet came in the form of three categories (protein, carbs and colour). Well, as luck would have it, I also have three categories for a varied, balanced exercise routine. They are: SWEAT, STRONG and SOOTHE. I'll explain them below.

NOTE: Many types of exercise are a mixture of two, or even three, of these. These kinds of exercises are brilliant multitaskers!

Sweat

These are the kinds of exercises that get your heart pumping, building your cardiovascular fitness and endurance. They're going to be especially helpful if you want to lose weight, but they're also important if you want to live longer and just be a mega-fit legend. Cardio exercise can be the scariest and hardest type of exercise to get into, since it can get you sweaty and breathless – feelings that can be uncomfortable at first, especially if you're not used to them. Running and cycling are the most obvious types of cardio (and we'll come back to running in more detail on page 111), but here are some other types you could try . . .

Spin classes. You sit on a stationary exercise bike, usually syncing up your moves to the beat of the music. Be like Penny – you might just love it.

Rowing machines. As well as being great cardio, these are excellent for building full-body strength. Bonus points if you can row an actual boat and not just a gym machine.

Cross-trainers. Found in any good gym, these nifty machines mimic running but without being so hard on your joints. Result.

Boxing. Packs a punch (literally). You can either do it on your own with a punching bag or join a class where you will do some high-octane choreographed punches. It's fun AND a great release for any negative, angry energy.

Trampolining (or rebounding). Yes, jumping is a great form of cardio, and it's also really beneficial for circulation. Buy a mini rebounder for your garden or find a class near you.

Dance classes. Any kind of dance, whether Zumba or hip-hop (if you're feeling brave), is likely to get you sweating.

Hiking. Particularly if the terrain is uneven, or there's a hefty incline.

Step workouts. Using a raised platform (or step), these classes improve cardio health as well as build strength in your legs, glutes and core.

Strong

We've already touched on strength in Level 2 (and we'll come back to it in Level 5), so you don't need me to explain this one in too much detail. Strong workouts focus on your muscles and bones. Aesthetically, this kind of exercise is what tends to create that ripped or toned look (if that's what you're after), but most of all, it just props up your body and makes *everything* easier. Alongside bodyweight strength exercises you could also try . . .

Free weights. This is where you build your strength using dumbbells. All gyms will have a range of different weights, but you can also buy your own small dumbbells for effective home or garden workouts.

Kettlebell workouts. These involve holding a single weight that looks a bit like an old-fashioned kettle. Again, you can try these in the gym or buy some for home.

Resistance bands. These smart props add extra resistance (essentially, weight) to any body-weight exercises you do. We'll discuss these more in Level 5.

Barbell training. This involves using weights placed on either side of a bar to enhance results. They're often used for squats and chest presses. They're much less intimidating than they look, trust me.

Circuits. These classes involve rotating through strength workouts with minimal rest in between. The high intensity of the movements means they feel like cardio workouts, too! (We'll come back to these in Level 6.)

Reformer Pilates. Definitely not for the faint-hearted. These classes build strength and power, particularly in the core.

Soothe

These are the kinds of workouts where you don't have to go full-throttle – and that's intentional. You see, slowing down is actually vital for strengthening your heart and reducing injury, which helps to support all your other workouts. Not only that, these types of exercise are especially beneficial for their mood-boosting benefits, helping you to reset, recentre and stretch out both your muscles and your mind. That said, many of these exercises can still be bloody difficult, and can be classified as strength and/or cardio, if you increase the intensity. Besides long walks and standard yoga, here are some great soothing exercises you can try . . .

Swimming. It's an excellent form of cardio, but you're buoyed by the water so it's also good for relieving any tension in your muscles. Plus you can take it slow and float along if you like. Bliss.

Aqua aerobics. Strength-training and stretching moves, except in the water. Dreamy. I always recommend this to my older clients, as it's gentle on joints and bones.

Hot yoga. Yoga, but in hot rooms. These classes involve rolling out your mat in rooms that are heated to 35–40 degrees Celsius. The idea is to improve flexibility and circulation. Dynamic classes will feel more intense, while slower yin classes will feel more meditative – a bit like being in a sauna.

Barre. Combining elements of Pilates, yoga and ballet, these classes focus on strengthening and lengthening muscles. Both soothing and bloody challenging at the same time.

Aerial yoga. These classes involve performing yoga poses and moves while hanging from a giant piece of cloth, like a bat. If you've ever sought peace from hanging upside down, here is your chance!

Tai chi. This is a Chinese martial art that is used for health, relaxation and mindfulness rather than combat. It involves slow, flowing movements – no aggressive punches here.

TROTTER TASK: Create an exercise bucket list

Even if every single thing I mentioned above feels scary right now, I want you to write down a bucket list of classes or disciplines that you'd love to try. You don't have to like the look of everything, but I can guarantee at least a few of these exercises have caught your eye. If you love going to nightclubs, dancing might tickle your fancy. If you're into wellbeing and

---

mindfulness, aerial yoga or tai chi could be calling your name. Write your own personal bucket list here, and aim to tick off one type of exercise each month.

1 ....

2 ....

3 ....

4 ....

5 ....

Remember, if you're showing up to a class, gym or event to tick off your bucket list, own being a beginner. There's absolutely nothing wrong with it – everyone was a beginner at some point. Tell your instructor that it's your first session, and I can guarantee they'll make you feel comfortable in no time.

More ways to spice up your fitness life

There are so many different ways you can keep your workout routine feeling varied and exciting – even if you're more-or-less doing the same sessions and the same moves. Here are some ideas for your perusal . . .

Home versus gym

Some people are religious about doing either home workouts or going to the gym. Personally? I like to switch it up. Home workouts are great if you need to squeeze in something quick, but gym sessions are good for getting out of your usual headspace and absorbing the energised vibes of being in an environment designed specifically for fitness.

Indoors versus outdoors

This is such a great way to keep things interesting. When the sun's out, I like to take my mat outside and do some body-weight exercises, or even dumbbells. If it's cold and miserable, you could also try running on a treadmill inside instead of outside – this can be beneficial, as you control the conditions and you can adjust your incline and speed. (Cheeky hint: you can also watch your favourite Netflix show while you run – killing two birds with one stone.)

Solo workouts versus classes

You might view yourself as a lone ranger, and this can definitely be great for clearing your head and getting in the zone. But attending a class can make you feel part of a community, and allows you to follow along, rather than making decisions. Being on your own is meditative, while being in a group can be motivating. We'll get into group workouts more in Level 6.

Slow 'n' controlled versus hot 'n' heavy

Sometimes, you can do the exact same workout, just in a completely different way. For example, with a strength routine you could do fewer reps but keep them slower and controlled, taking breaks in between. Or you could move between them quickly, building up your stamina as you go. Both have their own benefits. Both are valid. Changing how you do the exact same routine is a supersonic way to keep things spicy.

FEAR: PREVENT INJURY

So many people are scared of exercising because they're anxious about getting injured. This is particularly true of my older clients, who worry that they'll twist or fall and do themselves some permanent damage.

Let's not beat around the bush here: it is absolutely possible to get injured while exercising. As we get older, our bodies *do* become more vulnerable to injury. Some injuries are completely out of our control, but when it comes to exercise, most of them are absolutely *within* our control. We can prevent and avoid them. All you need to do is make some simple injury-prevention tweaks to protect your muscles, nerves and bones.

Unfortunately, I had to learn this the hard way. You see, I was once the *opposite* of many of my fearful clients, in that I thought I was invincible when it came to exercise. I think that mindset came from the rugby field, where long-lasting injury simply *wasn't an option* if you wanted to stay on the team. If your knee or ankle hurt, you'd go to physio, strap it up, then get back on the field. As a result, I trained myself not to pay attention to any aches or niggles, thinking that it made me a 'strong' athlete to push through. It was a sort of 'keep calm and carry on' mentality.

As my social media following grew, I began taking on more and more exercise challenges, setting myself extremely difficult goals. I started being invited to compete in events – triathlons, half marathons, the lot – and I really struggled to say 'no'. I loved pushing myself, so I just thought, *Why the hell not?*

At that time, I probably needed someone to tap me on the shoulder and say: 'Buddy, if you keep pushing at this intensity, something's gonna give.' Although, to be honest, I probably would've ignored them anyway. Rather than resting after these big events, I'd throw myself straight into training for the next challenge, never giving my poor body a chance to catch a break.

Eventually, the pains came, but I still thought I could do some physio and get back to it. It was different every day, sometimes I felt completely fine, other days it was my knees, and on others, my hamstrings. That half marathon where I limped to the finish line was a wakeup call that I needed to properly address what was going on in my body. An MRI revealed that it was a complex spinal injury causing everything. I had caused it by pushing so hard for so long. And if I pushed any harder, I could risk doing permanent damage.

I'm not telling you this to scare you; I'm telling you this because it could so easily have been avoided if I wasn't such a silly sausage who got obsessed with crossing finish lines in record time. Looking back, there were so many warning signs, so many aches and pains, but I just kept on ignoring them. You can easily avoid this by staying in tune with your body, by listening to the feedback it's giving you. If something hurts, it's not a failure – it's a message.

So long as you prioritise balance over burnout, you can protect your body from over-strain. Not only that, there are so many things you can do to prevent injury – from warming up and cooling down correctly, to maintaining proper form in whatever you do.

But before we get into these tips and tricks, I want to remind you that exercise is still the best way of protecting your body against the knocks that life brings. Studies have found that exercise is one of the best ways of reducing the risk of falls and injury in later life – since balance and strength are cornerstones of longevity. *Not exercising* is more likely to lead to injury than exercising. If you have creaky bones and weak muscles, you're more likely to fall and hurt yourself, and if you're not healthy in body and mind, it could take you a lot longer to recover from an injury. My mum, who broke her shoulder falling off her bike, knows this all too well. The strength and fitness she had built up before her injury undoubtedly shortened her recovery time. What a hero.

So, you see, exercise-related injury shouldn't hold you back from doing it. Just follow my tips below and you'll protect your body as much as possible.

Walk before you run

Having read Level 1 already, I hope you are already doing this – but here's another reminder. You don't need to (and shouldn't) dive headfirst into fast running, heavy weights and advanced moves without any prior training. Going at your own pace not only sets you up to succeed, it also protects your body from being shocked. If you suddenly turn on muscles that have never been used before, of course it's gonna hurt. My mum took this advice perfectly. When she started getting into workouts, she began with jogs that progressed into runs. She started with bodyweight that progressed into heavier weight. She kept taking baby steps along her journey, and she slowed down and went backwards a little if something felt too difficult. Even with the exercises I suggest in this book, it's okay if they feel too hard and you need to modify them or take it easier. It's not a failure – it's you priming your body to get the most out of exercise without shocking your system, which also means you're less likely to hurt yourself.

Always warm up and cool down

I know, I know. Sometimes you want to just get straight to it and then get back to your day when you're done. But trust me, it pays to warm up and cool down. If you jump straight into intense exercise it can lead to strains, sprains or even worse injuries, which is why it's so important to get your body ready for your workout. Likewise, cooling down with some gentle stretches can help prevent muscle soreness, as well as maintain healthy blood flow.

Your warm-ups and cool-downs will probably look different depending on what kind of exercise you're doing, but the trick is to do a warm-up that slightly mimics the moves you're going to do in your main workout, and a cool-down that stretches out the muscles you worked the most. But if you're not sure, here are a couple of one-size-fits-all warm-ups and cool-downs you can fall back on. I have made them each five minutes long because this is usually enough for me. However, spend as much time as you need warming up and cooling down. I know some people who spend 20 minutes warming up – and good on 'em.

THE 5-MINUTE WARM-UP

Perform each move for 45–50 seconds.

Jogging on the spot. Lift your knees up towards your chest. You should start to feel warmer and more mobilised very quickly.

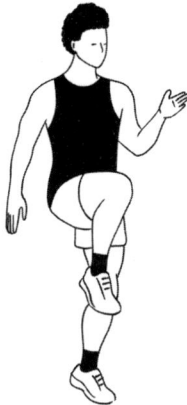

Slow reverse lunges. Step one leg back, lower yourself down, then return to standing. Repeat, alternating your legs. (See page 48.)

Side lunges. Step to the side and bend one knee while keeping the other leg straight. Keep your chest lifted and your hips back. Stick to one side for 25 seconds, then repeat on the other side.

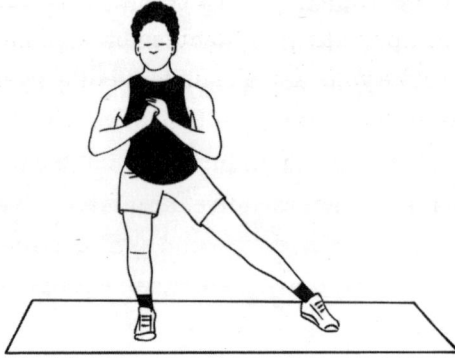

Toe touch to overhead reach. Slowly bend down to touch your toes (or shins) while keeping your legs straight. Roll up through your spine and reach your arms overhead for a slight stretch in your back. This will help your spinal mobility and your hamstrings.

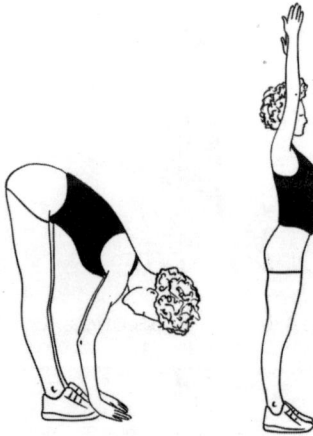

Walk-outs. From standing, fold forward, then walk your hands into a high plank. Pause there briefly, then walk your hands back and stand up. This warms up your shoulders, core and stretches those hamstrings. (See page 46.)

Greatest stretch of all time. So-called because it just feels *so good*. From a lunge position with your right leg back, plant down your right hand and rotate your left arm up to the sky. Then shift your weight back to stretch the front leg's hamstrings. Keep alternating between sides.

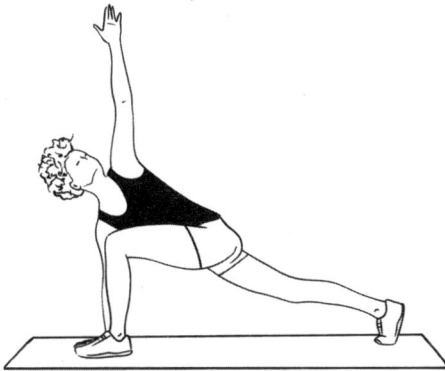

Call on your unicorn. Shout: 'Unicorn, I'm ready for you!!!' (optional).

THE 5-MINUTE COOL-DOWN

Try to hold each stretch for 30–60 seconds, focusing on deep and slow breathing.

Cross-body shoulder stretch. Bring one arm across your chest. Use the opposite hand to press the arm into your body. Keep your shoulders relaxed. This is great for upper-body workouts, or anything that might have fatigued your posture. Switch sides after around 30 seconds.

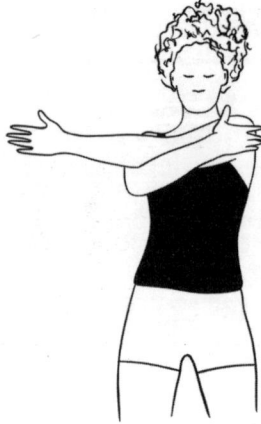

Standing figure-four stretch. Standing tall, cross one ankle over the opposite knee. Sink your hips back into a gentle squat, like you're sitting in a chair. Place your hands on your heart or resting on your standing leg for stability. This is great for your hips and glutes. Switch sides after 30 seconds.

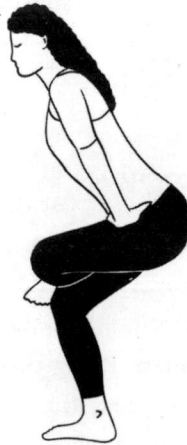

Seated hamstring stretch. Sit with one leg extended and the other bent in. Reach towards your extended foot, keeping your spine as straight as possible. Inhale to lengthen and exhale to deepen the stretch. Switch sides after 30 seconds.

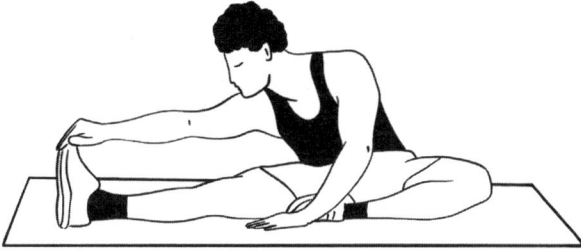

Lying supine twist. Lie on your back, bringing your knees over to one side, with your arms out wide on either side. Gaze in the opposite direction to your knees. You might want to hold your hips with the opposite arm for support. Switch sides after 30 seconds.

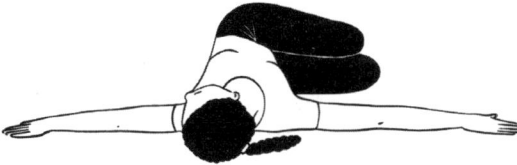

Toe touch to overhead reach. Repeat this move that you already did in your warm-up, except focus more on your breathing this time. Inhale as you reach overhead, and exhale as you reach down to touch your toes. Take your time, slowly make the move over 60 seconds. On your final roll-down, take a big sigh out of your mouth and give yourself a little round of applause as you roll up, for completing your workout. (See page 106.)

Invest in appropriate kit

The right kit can make all the difference in supporting your body through movement. If you're keen to get into running, I'd highly recommend buying your trainers from a specialist running shop and asking them to check your gait (which is basically *how* you run), as this can ensure you choose the right shoes for you. Shorts and sports bras that are supportive and don't chafe can also be really important. What's comfortable for 1 metre might not be so comfy for a 5k. Test everything out and make adjustments if you need to.

Prioritise proper form

Whatever exercise you're doing, proper form is *so* important. What this means is you're in the correct position, which means you are activating the correct muscles intended for that specific move. If you don't adopt the correct position (for example, if you're too hunched over in a squat, or you're tensing your neck, or you're not activating your core in Pilates), this can lead to strain and injury in body parts that have no business even being *involved* with that move. Even the most experienced athletes (ahem, me) can make mistakes with their form. When I was diagnosed with my spiral injury, I learned that I had been running all wrong. I had run a marathon in under 3 hours, so I assumed my running was perfect, but the truth is, my cadence was low, meaning my feet weren't hitting the floor enough, and they were taking a lot of impact that eventually aggravated my spine. The best way to avoid issues with your form? Speak to a personal trainer, if you can, or even ask for help from someone who knows. There's no shame in asking for help – in fact, there's power in it, because correcting your form will not only enhance your results, it'll also keep your body safe.

Listen to pain

Pain exists to tell you something – so make sure you bloody well listen. This doesn't mean you need to stop exercising because of any type of pain, it just means you need to tune in and listen, then adapt accordingly. For example, after completing a work-out (particularly if you're activating muscles for the first time in a while, or maybe even ever) you're likely to experience muscle soreness over the next few days. This is called DOMS – Delayed Onset Muscle Soreness. It's a completely normal part of exercising, and I sometimes feel a bit of pride when the DOMS sets in and I struggle to sit down on the loo, because it shows I was giving my muscles some attention. However, you can still listen to that pain. If you have intense DOMS in your legs, you might want to focus your next workout on your upper body so you don't aggravate that pain – or opt for something like swimming (check out the 'soothe' category on page 98). You don't have to push through DOMS, but you don't have to suffer through it either.

However, the types of pains that happen *when* you're exercising – a twinge in your hip or a creak in your knee – should never be ignored. If your body is shouting at you during your workout, stop what you're doing and try something else. Don't ignore it. Likewise, if the pain after your workout feels different to DOMS and is genuinely preventing you from doing normal movements, like walking or reaching – trust yourself and trust your body. Make sure you rest, and/or book in with a physio. Listen to your body, because it almost *always* knows when something needs to change.

FITNESS: RUNNING

There's a reason why, on a Sunday morning, you'll see every Tom, Dick and Harry out running around your local park. It's because running is one of the best forms of exercise you can do. It's the most accessible – you don't need a gym membership, and you can literally do it anywhere. It's also extremely tough – physically and emotionally. There's nowhere to hide when you're running. You have to keep pushing forward. It requires a lot of strength and a lot of resilience. It can be bloody difficult, but it's also really rewarding. The feeling you get after finishing a run is called 'Runner's High' – a rush of endorphins that genuinely feels like you've taken some kind of drug (I wouldn't know anything about that, mind you). It's true, you can get a high after most kinds of exercise, but I promise there's nothing like the high you get from running.

When I had to stop running for six months thanks to my spinal injury, I found it so difficult. I really missed the sense of escape it gave me, the whoosh of speed I felt flying through the air, the strength building in my calves and thighs, the blast of music in my ears. Those who get it, *get it*. And those who don't get it, *you can and will get it*. You just have to give it a go.

I know running might not seem like the most welcoming space. With so much focus on races and marathons, it might seem like an exclusive club that only the very fast and very fit are welcomed into. But that's truly far from reality. What I love most about running is that it's for everyone, and race days are full of people of all different backgrounds, shapes, sizes and speeds, united by their love of the run. Some people run purely because they want to get fit. Some people run because it helps them process grief or sadness, or it allows them to address their demons. Some people run because they have a goal in mind, and they love the sense of challenge and reward. Some people run simply because their friends do, and they enjoy the takeaway coffee at the end. Everyone runs for different reasons, and everyone is welcome. You don't have to be initiated into a club to be called a runner. If you run, you're a runner. Simples.

So if you're ready to give it a go (and lemme tell you, you are!), here are my top tips for joining the Runner's High Fanbase.

Check your gait. I already mentioned this on page 110, but this reminder is really important when you get into running. Most running stores can help with this – they have special equipment that can check the pattern of how your feet land on the floor when you run, offering advice about the right trainers and also how to make adjustments for your own safety. But it's important to note that everyone looks a little different when they're running – and it's okay if your style of running differs slightly from your mate's. We're all on our own journeys!

Invest in running kit (if you can). I have already spoken about the importance of good kit, but I think with running it's especially beneficial for the *intention* it sets. You'll need the right pair of trainers for you, leggings/tops that don't ride up or down with movement and that will dry up sweat (trust me), and ideally a running vest so you can easily carry water (and your phone). It's true, you can run with the bare minimum of kit, but I think you're more likely to enjoy and embrace running if you have comfortable kit that you really like. If you had a banged-up car, you'd be less careful with nicking it, but if you had an expensive car (or just one you love), you'd be really careful with it. The same goes with your kit. When you make the investment, you're more likely to treat the pursuit of running with respect.

Increase gradually. There are so many brilliant running apps out there – from Couch to 5k for beginners, to Runna for more advanced training plans. The whole idea is that they take the guesswork out of how and when to increase your distance, which is super helpful. It's totally fine to start with extremely short runs (even 1k), and also to break up your runs into walking and running intervals. There's no shame in starting somewhere. Keep that beginner's attitude in mind and you'll keep making improvements as you go along. You'll be running a marathon in no time! (Not that you *need* to . . . but you could.)

Know your route. Please, don't just leave your house with no idea of your direction or route. I'd recommend researching a route in advance – or it might be as easy as just doing laps of your local park. For safety reasons, you might want to choose a well-lit, well-trodden path, or you could go down quieter roads if you'd prefer to avoid crowds. Map out your route before you start so you don't have to think about it when you're pounding the pavements.

Aim for steady state. This essentially means you're doing a consistent, moderately paced run that you can sustain for a longer period without getting out of breath. Often, there's a temptation to try to run like the wind, but this is generally unsustainable (especially without much experience) and you're likely to burn out and run out of energy quickly. Pace yourself. Go slowly. You're not trying to beat anyone. Remember, it's you versus you. And anyway, steady, slow running can actually help you reduce your heart rate, which is needed if you ever want to take on bigger challenges (because lower heart rate = your body isn't working as hard). It's a very smart way to move.

Don't take running too seriously. It doesn't need to be a form of punishment. You can enjoy your runs more by blasting some of your favourite music, listening to a comedy podcast, or even playing little games with yourself like counting and noticing things in your surroundings. Running outside and in nature is really quite wonderful for your mental health, especially if you're able to run in green spaces or near water. Stop and take pictures. Maybe even have a little cry about how beautiful the world is. When you feel connected to nature, you feel happier. And that's a fact.

Focus on feelings, not times. It's easy to track your progress in running – you can see if you've increased your speed or distance easily with some kind of smartwatch. But progress can also come in the form of *feeling better about running*. It doesn't matter if you haven't shaved a second off your usual time and you're running the exact same route – if you're enjoying it more, then you're on the up. Celebrate every milestone, no matter how small. We'll come back to this idea, and the pros and cons of tracking exercise, in Level 5.

CAN'T RUN?

If you're injured, or your doctor has advised against running for whatever reason, cycling is a great cardiovascular alternative. You get a lot of the same benefits – being outside, feeling the wind in your hair (or beard) and building strength and improving your heart health, without such heavy impact on your joints. Just make sure you prioritise safety – always wear a helmet, maintain your bike and only cycle on terrain and at speeds you feel comfortable with.

FUN: CASH-IN YOUR CARDIO

If the endorphin rush after your cardio sesh wasn't enough, a rewards system is bound to make it a lot more fun and exciting. With this challenge, every improvement you make in either distance or time warrants some kind of prize. And who doesn't like winning prizes?! (In fact, we'll be getting into this in more detail in the next Level).

This isn't a race in the traditional sense – it's only you versus you, and you're completely capable of winning. Every time you show up, you build strength, confidence and consistency. Choose your pace, strap in and earn those rewards.

First, choose your cardio toy. If you want to stick to outdoor running or cycling, that's fine, too, but you can also opt for a treadmill, an exercise bike, a cross-trainer or a rowing machine. Whatever excites you and makes you feel your best. If you're going to run or cycle outdoors, though, I'd suggest having some kind of watch so that you can track your distance and time (most machines in a gym will do this for you).

Next, choose your distance or time. Over the course of a few weeks, you'll be increasing either your time (how long you spend doing this type of cardio), or your distance (how many kilometres you cover over the course of the week). You might prefer to choose time if you want something flexible and with less pressure – you can reduce your effort levels, as long as you clock in those minutes or hours. If you want a greater challenge, you might want to choose distance, which can help you build endurance. However, both of them will pack a punch, so go with whatever feels right for you.

If you're increasing time . . .

Week 1 – 60 minutes total (e.g. 3 x 20 minutes)

Week 2 – 90 minutes total

Week 3 – 110 minutes total

Week 4 – 130–150 minutes total

If you're increasing distance . . .

Week 1 – 5km total

Week 2 – 7.5km total

Week 3 – 10km total

Week 4 – 12–15km total

Treat yourself

If you manage to hit your target each week, WELL BLOODY DONE. But don't just let my congratulations be your sole reward. You deserve a treat every time you reach your new goal. Here are some ideas for ways to cash-in your cardio.

Week 1 – Buy yourself a fancy coffee, your favourite picky bits from M&S, or light the expensive candle you've been saving for a special occasion. You showed up! You deserve it!

Week 2 – Time to indulge in some pampering. Take a 20-minute bubble bath, use a face mask or take a guilt-free nap. Whatever a bit of peace means to you.

Week 3 – Completed almost two hours of cardio? Nothing sexier. Treat yourself to something that makes you feel SEXY! New skincare, some brand-new undies, or even a bottle of your favourite wine.

Week 4 – You made it! Now you get to cash-in your best reward. A solo adventure, a date night, a spa sesh or new gym gear. Whatever screams 'yep, I *did* the damn thing'.

If it takes you a little longer to get through the challenge than four weeks, that's totally fine too. You still deserve a reward each time you hit those markers. You're galloping on that unicorn – and it's truly a sight to see.

STAY ON TRACK

FOCUS: TRACK YOUR PROGRESS

Gone are the days of winging it. In this strange ol' world we live in, technology means that pretty much *everything* can be measured and tracked – from how many litres of water you drink in a day to the length of your periods (if you have them). And nowhere is our obsession with counting and storing data more obvious – and more used – than in the fitness space.

Fitness trackers and smartwatches are absolutely everywhere. In fact, recent research suggested that one in five people in the UK own a smartwatch (but I reckon this is even higher now).[1] I understand why people like them so much. For starters, you can track so many different measurements. You can track the number of steps you take per day, which is brilliant because research suggests that 8,000–10,000 steps per day can reduce the risk of illness and increase lifespan.[2] Knowing how many steps you're getting (and increasing them wherever possible) can be a really useful metric to measure.

---

1 https://www.lboro.ac.uk/research/climb/news/2024/blogwearabletech nology/

2 https://jamanetwork.com/journals/jamanetworkopen/fullarticle/280 2810

Then there are so many stats you can measure while you're working out. When running or cycling, you can easily track your distance and your speed (which will be particularly helpful if you have goals in mind, like the challenge you just completed in Level 4). You can also track how many kilocalories you burn per workout session (useful if you're trying to lose weight), plus your heart rate – the lower it is during movement, the fitter you're getting.

And beyond only tracking movement, you can also track your recovery. New trackers like Whoop, alongside traditional smartwatches, place a big emphasis on tracking sleep and downtime, giving 'readiness' scores and making sure you're also looking after your body *in between* those workout sessions.

If you find a fitness tracker helpful, I think that's bloody fantastic. I don't blame you at all – in the past, I have been rather in love with my Garmin watch (heart-eye emoji). When I had a specific goal in mind – like running a marathon in under three hours – my watch was the guiding light I needed to track my progress. I could see, very easily, if my splits were improving enough to reach that very specific time I was aiming for. I probably couldn't have done it without my watch, giving me the real shiny hard data to know I was moving forward.

However, as we all know by now, my fitness goals involved pushing my body to my limit – and that didn't work out so well for me and the ol' spine in the long run. So, now I think, was it *really* such a good thing to have focused so heavily and obsessively on the numbers? In hindsight, I'm not so sure.

You see, whenever I hit a new time or distance, *that's* what became my baseline. Even though it was bloody hard and really impressive to reach that target, and I should've celebrated being a fitness legend, it suddenly became my 'default' – something I needed to beat and push past. From that point on, anything that fell short of the number I had achieved was considered a let-down.

It wasn't *entirely* the tracker's fault. Yes, it gave me the numbers. But it was *me* who allowed those numbers to push me into burnout. I thought this was a sign of strength – that I was highly motivated, passionate and ambitious. And, yes, I was. But my body eventually paid the price.

A similar thing happened to one of my friends, Jake*. Except his tracking obsession came in the form of sleep. He had a demanding job that meant waking up early in the mornings, and he knew he functioned better if he had eight hours of solid sleep. So he started tracking his sleep to ensure he was going to bed on time, getting sufficient amounts of REM and deep sleep (the amounts you need to properly recover – which we'll come back to in Level 7), in a bid to wake up feeling more refreshed. So far, so fair. But this all went a bit wrong when he started becoming really anxious in the evenings, worried that if he didn't get to sleep bang on time, his next day would suffer and he'd fail at work. This became a vicious cycle – the anxiety got in the way of his sleep, and when he woke up the next morning to lower numbers, he felt *even worse*.

He thought the tracking was helping him, but actually it was worsening the problem. It added fuel to the fire, giving him something to obsess over, and making sleep a source of stress – when that's the *opposite* of what sleep is all about. Eventually, he realised that this was the issue, switched off his sleep tracking and removed some of the pressure. And guess what? His sleep became more restful, more consistent and easier to come by.

I'm not saying that tracking has this effect on everyone. I'm saying it's really important to be mindful of whether your tech is helping you stick to your goals or adding unnecessary pressure and obsession that you could just do without. Remember: we're all different. Just because it works for your mate doesn't mean it will work for you. If you are already using a watch, and you're not sure if it's your friend or your foe, here are some signs to look for . . .

DATA TRACKING: FRIEND	DATA TRACKING: FOE
You enjoy checking your times/distances/numbers – they give you a boost and generally make you feel good about yourself.	You dread checking your data and find that it generally makes you feel deflated and discouraged.
If your numbers drop for whatever reason, you take it all in your stride and use it as motivation for next time.	If your numbers drop, you use this as a reason to beat yourself up and get down on yourself.
You can go without checking your data – you don't look at it obsessively. You only check it whenever it feels relevant and useful.	You obsessively keep tabs on your data and find yourself adapting your lifestyle to meet your goals (for example, walking around the block 10 times at midnight to meet your step target).
You get a sense of reward and satisfaction out of seeing your numbers climb and your targets being hit.	Any reward you feel for achieving your goals is quickly overshadowed by a feeling of 'what next?'

If you want to start (or continue) tracking your workouts using a digital tracker or smartwatch – I salute you, my friend. But just keep an eye on this chart. Your tracker should be there to encourage you, support you and motivate you with your goals. If it keeps you consistent and excited about exercising, then it's absolutely a positive thing. But if your tracker begins to feel more like a foe than a friend, it could be time to break up with it – or at least monitor how you're using these metrics. There are ways you can stop the numbers from dominating how you feel – like removing certain metrics from your app homepage, or turning off notifications.

Whatever you decide, your watch, ring or other kind of tracker doesn't need to be the be-all and end-all. You can track your progress in other ways.

Tracking feelings, not numbers

My injury gave me much more of a level head about my targets and goals. I still think it's important to feel like you're constantly improving and getting better, because this is absolutely key to maintaining both motivation and discipline. When we feel like we're succeeding, this gives us even more fuel *to* succeed. When we feel like our hard work is paying off, we're more likely to work even harder. But we can't base our improvements solely on numbers on a screen or a scale. My new motto is 'My personal best isn't a time or a distance, it's a *feeling*'.

I'm working towards that sense of reward on the other side of achieving something difficult. It doesn't matter if I cycled slower. It doesn't matter if I've gained a bit of weight here or there. If I'm feeling as good as I possibly can, that's progress, baby! Numbers are useful, but they don't tell the whole story.

'But Tommy, how can you measure feelings instead of times or distances? I don't have that function on my smartwatch!'

I know, I know. The best way to do this is by having check-ins with yourself after every workout sesh. Ask yourself the following questions, ranking them on a scale of 1–10: 1 being not very much, 10 being *very*.

- How strong do I feel?
- How capable do I feel?

- How agile (quick and responsive) do I feel?
- How energised do I feel?

If your numbers are increasing after every sesh, then, jeepers creepers, you're progressing marvellously! But if you find the numbers fluctuating a little, it doesn't mean you're going backwards, it just means every day is different. We all have days where we're in a funk, we're tired, or we could be affected by illness or hormones (if you have menstrual cycles, you might notice a little backward roll in the days leading up to your period). It's totally okay for your scores to jump around and go up and down. It's all about the general progression over time. If you're gradually working your way up that scale, then you're doing something right.

Every time you fill in these check-ins, notice the sense of pride that rises up within you. That's the roar of a lion, my friend. That's a sense of achievement you deserve to celebrate.

More ways to track progress

As much as feelings are the priority, I also think it can be helpful to track milestones as you go along. Whether that's completing more than an hour's worth of exercise in a week, finally reaching that 5k, or working up to 10kg dumbbell weights. Tracking (and celebrating) these milestones will motivate you to move on to the next one and prevent you from staying stranded at one level in your training. That's the whole point of this book, isn't it? Gradually working your way up to get fitter, stronger, healthier and happier.

Hopefully you've already completed (or are working on) the Fun section from Level 4, which was all about rewards, and hopefully you've noticed just how *damn good* those rewards felt. This is because humans are simple creatures, and we *love* rewards. In science speak, this is called 'positive reinforcement'. You might know about this phrase if you've ever trained a dog. Lots of dog trainers use treats to help dogs behave better – every time they exhibit some good-boy (or girl) behaviour, they get a treat. Humans aren't so different.

The more positivity we receive from doing something, the more we feel motivated to keep going back and doing it again and again.

That's because something amazing happens in the brain when we receive a reward or treat. We get a hit of dopamine, which is a neurotransmitter associated with happiness and pleasure. We already experience a rush, or high, once we've exercised, since we get flooded with endorphins, but adding in a reward can be even more enjoyable and satisfying. It feels like we're 'winning' something – a bit like playing a game. And who doesn't love a game?!

You can create positive reinforcement to track your progress really easily. You don't need physical and tangible rewards (like you had in the Cash-In challenge on page 115) to feel the benefits. It can be as simple as any one of these suggestions below.

A habit tracker. You simply tick off every time you exercised in a given week. Rather than focusing on time, distance or weight goals, this is simply a visual representation of your ability to stay committed and consistent, which is great for the ol' self-esteem, and will encourage you to keep going. Here's an example of how to make one. You can colour (or draw an X, or whatever you fancy) in the box whenever you complete that exercise. Looking at empty boxes isn't so satisfying – so you'll want to fill in those bad-boys!

	M	T	W	T	F	S	S
WEIGHTS		X					
RUNNING	X				X		
YOGA				X			X

A list on your fridge of all your goals. This can be the weights you want to achieve, distances to run, etc. – whatever metrics you want to track. Then tick them off each time you achieve one. Even the small act of ticking something off activates that reward centre in the brain and releases dopamine. Having this visual representation of what you've already achieved can be mega inspiring.

A star-chart. Instead of ticks you can use shiny, gold, star-shaped stickers. Yes, just like you might make for children! We are all big kids deep down, and if you remember how good it felt to have a chart full of stars (and a reward at the end of it), then why not create one for yourself? There ain't nothing wrong with bringing out your inner child.

A money jar or piggy bank. Drop in a pound every time you finish a workout or reach a goal. Once again, who said piggy banks are just for kids? *Boring!!* Maybe you have a treat goal in mind – an item of clothing, a spa day or a piece of furniture you want to buy that feels like too much of a treat. This way, you will *literally* earn that treat. Listening to the clink of adding more coins to the bank – instant gratification. You also have the double benefit of working towards greater health *and* something luxurious.

A visual thermometer or progress bar for a specific goal. Make this something achievable, such as running 15k. Colour it in as you get more kilometres under your belt, so you can see just how close you are to reaching that goal. Watching the tank 'filling up' will help you fill up your energetic tank, too.

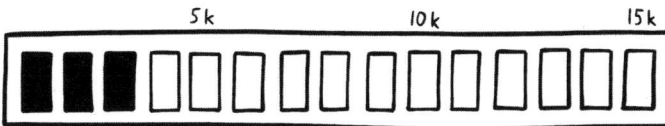

Progress pictures. If your aim is to lose weight or change your body composition, this can be a helpful approach to track how your body is changing. Take pictures in the mirror after every workout, adopting the same stance and ideally wearing the same clothes. Over time, you'll see your body changing. My clients know how bloody inspiring this can be – their before and after pics are mega! However, remember that you're unlikely to notice physical changes within the first couple of months – you have to be locked in and still committed to the long game, so it's helpful to track like this in tandem with another form of progress-tracking. Remember: aesthetics are only one part of the story.

The choice is yours

Yep, I'm a broken record, but I'm gonna say it again: this is your journey. You get to decide the metrics you measure (distance, time, feelings or even just showing up). You get to decide how you track them. You get to decide if you even want to track them *at all.* Some people enjoy the sense of reward while others find it too much pressure. Personally, I think there's some way of tracking for everyone, you just have to find what works for you. Because when you see how much progress you're making, you feel motivated to keep doing more. When you see how far you've come, you feel confident in your own ability to push yourself to move forward. You become your own fitspiration. You become more proud of yourself than ever before. As you bloody well should!

FEAR: HOLD YOURSELF ACCOUNTABLE

There's a reason why my coaching biz just keeps growing and growing. It's not because I'm a charming, good-looking, hilarious chap (although maybe a little), it's because fitness coaching fills a void that so many people need. It's perfect for people who need someone else to hold them accountable.

So, what do I mean by accountability? It's basically about having that tap on the shoulder – from something or someone – that says: 'Here's what you need to do. You've got this. I believe in you. Keep going.' Accountability keeps you on your 'why' path. It helps you maintain your structure and discipline. It reminds you to push through failures and keep going even when the going gets tough. Accountability encourages you to show up, but it also encourages you to *push yourself* when you're there and get the best out of every workout.

For many of my clients, they need some external accountability – meaning, *someone else* who can hold their hand through the whole process. This is usually because they have tried exercising in other ways – signing up to a gym, downloading a home-workout app, buying some equipment – but it just doesn't stick. This isn't because they don't have a why. It's not because they are totally undisciplined and lack organisation. It's just that they need that companion who can keep them on the straight and narrow, reminding them of their purpose, their resilience, their goals. Because, quite honestly, it's very easy to forget.

This is why my client, Mo*, finally reached out to me – after months of deliberating – on a sunny April morning. Every single January, without fail, he had set the intention that *this* would be the year he got in shape. He had a clear why: he wanted to play football with his sons and not be left wheezing. He wanted to get back to the sporty, athletic guy he was at university – which is where he met his wife – and he remembered this time fondly as his most confident years. He knew *how* to exercise (as this was his passion when he was young) and he also had some time to exercise, since he mostly worked in the mornings, so generally had the afternoons off. There was, really, no reason why he shouldn't be able to stick to his exercise regime. Except . . .

His mind often got in the way. When he didn't see results straight away, he wondered if it was even possible for him to return to his former glory. His wife and kids didn't seem to particularly care whether he worked out or not – and often encouraged him to join them in front of the TV when he was just about to head to the gym. Each and every time, his why became too distant and his discipline faltered. And that's when he decided he needed some outside help.

It's a completely natural thing to need. There's no shame in needing support from someone, or something, else. Whether you want kindness or a kick up the backside, sometimes the biggest difference between sticking with it, and not sticking with it, is having someone hold you accountable. My job, as a coach, is to make things really easy for my clients, to guide them through the process and to remind them why they're here to begin with. It's not about me or my goals or what I want – it's my job to keep them coming back to the path they *want* to travel but struggle to stick to.

This is what happened with Mo. Whenever he felt his motivation slowly slipping away, I was there on the other end of the phone saying, 'Get yourself to that workout. Gallop on that unicorn! You've got this!' And what person in their right mind would say no to that?! Coaching is really simple when you think about it, but it's so effective. It means many of my clients can relax into knowing that someone has their back. Someone is looking out for their best interests. Someone *knows* why they're here and wants to see them achieve their goals. This was the first time Mo ever stuck to exercising for more than two months. What a hero.

External accountability comes in lots of different forms. You might not always get it from a coach like me. You can get it from a personal trainer who pushes you in your sessions to work harder than you ordinarily would on your own. You can get it from your Pilates instructor, who tells you to do just *one more leg-raise* even when you feel like your bum might fall off. It might even be your partner, who will kick you to get up for your alarm and go work out, even when you really, really want to sleep in peace. Maybe it's even an app on your phone that dings reminders and words of encouragement. You could even use an AI bot to chivvy you along. They won't be quite as good as a real-life coach, but something could be better than nothing.

I strongly recommend you find someone or something to hold you accountable, particularly when you're in your earliest stages of exercising. Sometimes, all you need is to feel like someone else *cares* about your journey (even if that someone is an app or a robot) – as this will make you care about your own progress even more.

External accountability can play such an important role in exercising, but it really shouldn't last forever. Eventually, all my clients end up flying the nest. They take the accountability I provide and then they learn how to be those accountable cheerleaders *for themselves*. They don't need me anymore. My work is done.

After several months, Mo decided that it was time to branch out on his own. He knew what he was doing, and he had accumulated all the skills he needed to become his own pep-talker. He became accountable to himself. Essentially, he could motivate himself to keep going, he could convince himself to push harder. He became that steady, reassuring, helpful voice seeing him through each workout. It didn't happen overnight, but internal accountability took over as his primary source of accountability.

When your inner voice is the loudest motivating voice, then you know you're fully in the groove.

'So, how do you build internal accountability?' I hear you ask. Well, if you've been working through these levels, you've already started doing it. If you're constantly reminding yourself of your why, you're holding yourself accountable. If you're working hard to overcome fear of failure and push through setbacks, you're holding yourself accountable. If you have created a clear structure and routine, you're holding yourself accountable. Pushing yourself to stick to your habits and stay true to your goals is the *definition* of holding yourself accountable. But here are a few more things you can do to enhance that accountability and become your own personal fitness coach. Wallop!

Keep reviewing your structures. Putting a routine in place is the first sign of accountability. But you also need to keep reviewing these routines to make sure it's all still working for you. Could you, realistically, increase the amount of time you spend working out? Or maybe you need to reduce it, but to make up for that you could increase the intensity of your workouts. Don't be afraid to switch it up. If something about your routine is stopping you from operating at full capacity, it's totally okay to reassess.

TROTTER TASK: Give yourself an end-of-month review

Think of this as like having a review meeting with your boss . . . except your boss is you, and your job is being a fitness supremo. Answer the following questions:

What have I done well this month? (e.g. showed up to every workout, moved up a dumbbell bracket in weights workouts.)

What wasn't so good? (e.g. skipped a few workouts because of a hangover, losing motivation to run.)

What steps will I take to tackle any problems? (e.g. get stuff ready the night before, invite a friend to go running.)

What are my targets for next month? (e.g. try a new class, find cycling sessions easier.)

Create an alter-ego. If you really like the idea of having that external accountability coach, you can create an alter-ego who takes on that role. Give them a name (may I suggest: Tom Trotter), a personality (eccentric) and imagine the kinds of things they would say to you. Every time you consider skipping your workout or being a little lazy, imagine they're right there in the room with you. Think to yourself: 'What would Tom say right now?' Then give yourself that answer. You might even want to say the words aloud (if you're in a public space, just be aware you may look a little loco – I say, embrace it!).

Be really honest with yourself (like, *really* honest). Are you *really* skipping your workout today because you can't fit it in, or is it because you can't be bothered? Pay attention to the excuses you give yourself and know when you need a stern kick up the bum. This is what a coach would do – we're always kind, but we know when a bit of tough love is absolutely needed. Every time you want to make an excuse, visualise your imaginary coach shaking their head and saying, '*really?*' Sometimes we find it easier to lie to ourselves than we do to other people. If you look your alter-ego in the eyes, you might realise that you *should* be getting up for that workout, and you should be pushing yourself.

Give yourself pep-talks. I love a good pep-talk. There's something about a motivational speech that just makes me feel supported and unstoppable. It's nice to receive these from someone else, but it's not essential. I love to give pep-talks to myself, with video messages or voice memos, that I can return to again and again, and I highly recommend you do the same. The best pep-talks are tailored to you, they're reassuring, but tough. Here are some examples of phrases you can include in your own pep-talks, but follow your own instincts about what you find the most inspiring.

'I know you really don't feel like exercising right now, but *trust me*, you will feel so much better afterwards – you always do.'

'You are strong, you are capable, you have bloody well got this and I am so excited for you to reach all of your fitness goals.'

'Mate, I know you're struggling today, but I believe in you, you have made it through the worst struggles before, so you can damn well make it through this workout.'

You might think it's silly that the pep-talk is coming from yourself. But actually I think this is mega powerful.

Remember: *you* are the biggest cheerleader you could ever need.

Repeat affirmations. This is basically a quicker version of those pep-talks. Pick a few short phrases that resonate with you, and repeat them to yourself before your workouts, or during them, or afterwards, or whenever the hell you want really. You can say them in your head, or aloud (again, who cares what people think?!). Here are some examples . . .

'I am strong.'

'I am capable.'

'I can push myself.'

'I am resilient.'

'I am improving.'

'My hard work is paying off.'

Saying them over and over is like a mantra. Personally, I believe that you become your thoughts. You become what you tell yourself. Keep repeating these phrases to yourself, and eventually you'll believe them.

Forgive yourself. One big thing about having that coach alter-ego is that they are *separate to you*. This means they are likely to be kinder to you, more understanding, and, most importantly, they don't feel any shame on your behalf. Shame is a big word, isn't it? But so many of us feel it. Maybe you feel ashamed for going so long without exercising, or for not being as strong as you'd like, or for skipping a workout. But shame isn't going to help you in any way; all it does is make you feel more deflated and disheartened. And it's something we only ever project onto ourselves – you'd be very unlikely to feel ashamed of a mate for the same things. That's where your alter-ego comes in; they don't feel any shame about the times you slow down or give up; they can give you compassion and encourage you to come back even stronger next time.

FITNESS: LEVEL UP YOUR STRENGTH

In Level 2, we introduced strength-training using just your body weight. Now it's time to increase the stakes (and the weight). If you want to build strength long term, then using extra weight in your moves – and increasing that weight as you go along – is crucial. This is because your muscles respond well to stress. This means that when you lift something heavier than you're used to your muscle fibres will experience small amounts of damage. Don't worry, this isn't a bad thing – it signals to your body to re-build those fibres stronger and thicker than they were before, so that they're more able to handle a heavier weight next time. This is called progressive overload. It's how your muscles get stronger and stronger over time.

There are so many ways to encourage progressive overload in your own muscles. You can do this using handheld weights (like dumbbells and kettlebells), barbells and resistance bands (for more info on what each of these is and does, visit page 97). I want to start by talking you through some of the most useful gym machines, because I know they can look a bit intimidating if you have never done them before. Most of these machines work by using a stack of weights with various different weight bands – from light to heavy. You use a selector pin to choose which level of weight works for you. There's something really satisfying about returning to those same machines and noticing your pins get lower and lower, meaning you're performing the move with much more weight. Now *that's* a hit of dopamine if I've ever seen one!

Every time you use a machine, I recommend doing eight reps of that move. Repeat this four times with short breaks in between. Pick a weight that feels easy enough to do the first few but challenging towards the end. Gradually, your muscles adjust and it'll get easier to do the last few. That's when you know it's time to crank up the weight!

Remember, you probably won't be using an identical weight for each machine. We tend to find heavier weights easier when working our lower bodies (even for beginners), since we use our legs and glutes much more in everyday life than we do our backs, shoulders and arms. Don't be worried if you need a much lighter weight when working your upper body, that's totally normal.

Here are some of my favourite pieces of weighted gym equipment, and how to use them:

Leg press machine

Use for: Building strength in your glutes, hamstrings and quads. It's a bit like doing a squat, except you're more horizontal and it can feel safer and more controlled.

How to do it: Sit with your head and back against the pad on the machine and your feet flat on the foot plate. Select the weight that works for you using the pin (you can always adjust it if it feels too hard or too easy). Push the plate away by extending your legs, but don't lock your knees completely. Slowly bend your knees to return to home.

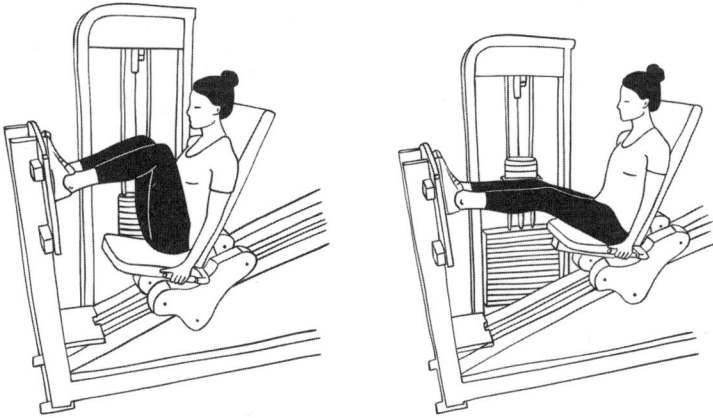

Chest press machine

Use for: Working your chest (pecs), triceps and shoulders.

How to do it: Sit with your back against the pad on the machine and hold onto the handles. Push forwards until your arms are extended (but not locked all the way). Slowly bring them back.

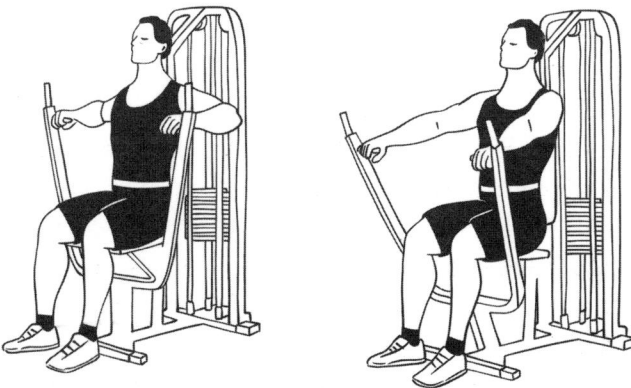

Lat pulldown machine

Use for: Strengthening your back, especially the V-shaped muscles in the centre.

How to do it: Sit with your thighs secure under the pad. Grab the bar, with your arms wider than your shoulders. Pull the bar down to your upper chest, squeezing your shoulder blades down and back. You should really be able to feel this in those back muscles. Then slowly return.

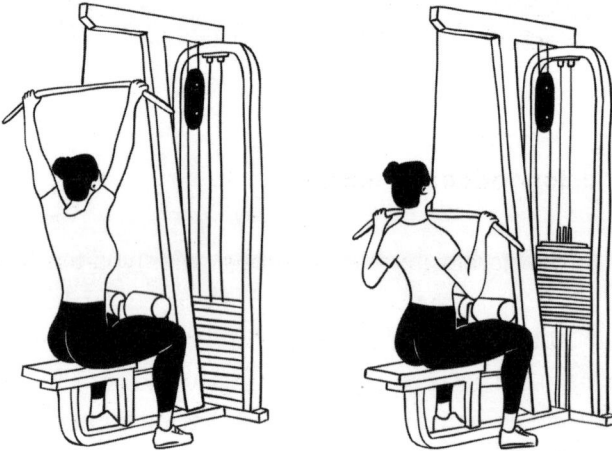

Leg extension machine

Use for: Working your quads (the muscles above your knees and in front of your thighs).

How to do it: Sit with the pad resting on your lower shins, select your weight, then gently extend your knees to lift the pad. Lower back down slowly. Try not to use this too extensively as it can stress the knees.

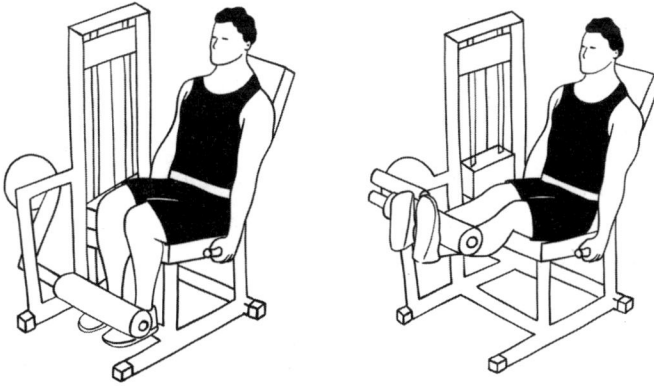

Hip abductor/adductor machine

Use for: Two different muscle isolations, when you use it in different ways. When you use it to push the legs out (abductor), this works the outer hip muscles. When you use it to push the legs in (adductor), it strengthens your inner thigh muscles.

How to do it (as an abductor): Sit with your back flat against the pad, with your thighs placed against the pads and your feet on the footrests. Select your desired weight with the pin, then push your legs outwards until you feel a squeeze in your outer hips. Then slowly return to the starting position.

How to do it (as an adductor): Sit on the machine with your back supported, except this time, place your feet on the outside of the pads. Most machines will have the option to flip the pads over and will have a different footrest position, so you'll still be comfortable using it in this way. Select the weight with the pin, then squeeze your legs together to bring the pads inward. Then slowly release back to your starting position.

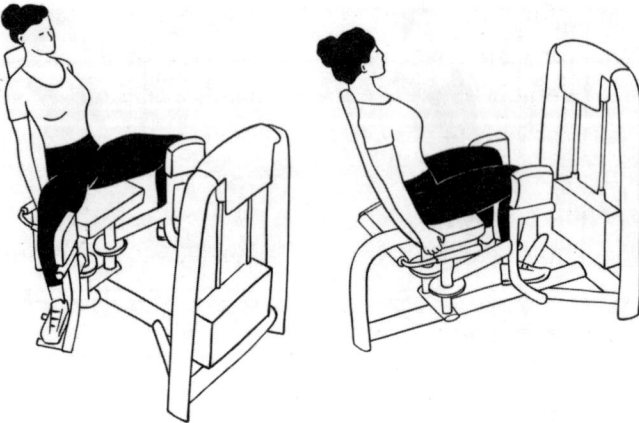

YOUR 20-MINUTE FULL-BODY DUMBBELL WORKOUT

Besides using the machines, free-weights like dumbbells are a great way to get that progressive overload going. This workout includes moves that focus on your whole body, so make sure to adapt the weight of your dumbbells as needed. You may need lighter for upper body and heavier for lower. It also includes compound exercises (moves that work multiple different muscle groups at the same time), which is a very efficient way of exercising.

Just like we mentioned with the weighted machines in the gym, it's important to choose your dumbbells wisely. Before you start, try lifting a very light weight. If it feels extremely easy for eight full reps, then it's too light for you. The perfect weight will feel manageable for the first few, but then the last couple of reps will feel like a challenge. Be realistic, it's totally okay if you start with a very light weight – even 1kg dumbbells are better than nothing! Once they start feeling easy the whole way through the reps, you know it's time to increase your weight (often after a couple of weeks of consistent movement).

It's also important to remember that you won't always use the same weight for different moves. You can usually handle heavier weights for your lower body, since these muscles tend to be stronger by default, as we use them much more. Don't be afraid to go lighter for your upper-body exercises, even the most experienced athletes will adapt their weights depending on which part of the body they are working!

This workout includes a warm-up, a main sesh, a core finisher and a cool-down. In the main sesh, spend 45 seconds doing each, then have a 15-second rest before moving on to the next move. Once you've finished all the moves, go back and repeat the whole thing a second time.

WARM-UP (2 minutes total)

Arm circles. (30 seconds) Simply hold out your arms and roll your shoulders in circles, making sure to change direction halfway through. Great for warming up the upper body.

Torso twists. (30 seconds) Twist your torso so that you look over your shoulders, back and forth on the left and right. Good for mobilising the spine and obliques.

Body weight squats. (30 seconds) With your feet hip distance apart, sit back as if you're sitting in a chair. This will warm up your lower body. We've done these before so you should be a pro by now!

Alternating lunges. (30 seconds) Again, we've done these before. From standing, reach one leg back into a lunge, then switch sides. Also great for warming up the lower body, plus it helps with your balance.

MAIN SESH (45 seconds for each move, 15 seconds rest.
Rest for 1 minute, then do another round – 12 minutes total)

Reverse lunges. Hold a dumbbell in each hand down by your hips, with arms straight. Step back into the lunge, pushing through the front heel to stand back up again. Keep alternating on both sides. (See page 48.)

Hammer curl into shoulder press. Curl your dumbbells up with your palms facing in, then lift (press) them above your head.

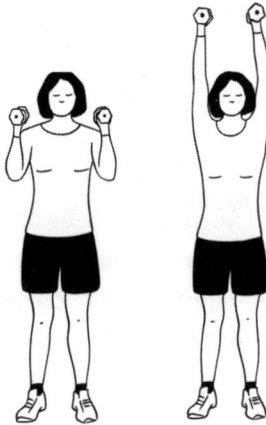

Thrusters. Holding your dumbbells up by your shoulders, drop down into a deep squat. Then push the dumbbells overhead on the way up. This is a superstar compound exercise.

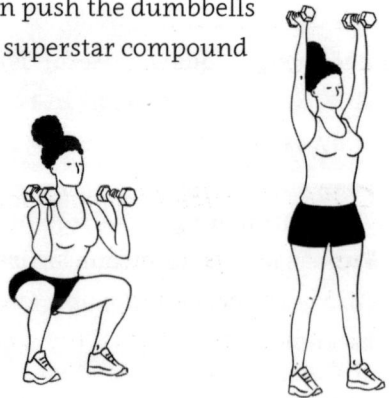

Lateral raises. Still holding a dumbbell in each hand, raise your arms sideways to shoulder height, pause, then bring them back down with control.

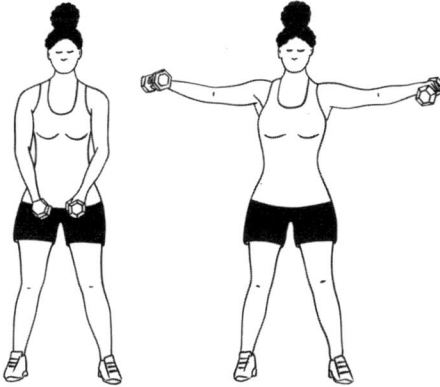

Dumbbell push-ups. Put your dumbbells down on the floor and grip both to keep your wrists neutral. With either your toes down or your knees down, lower your chest and then push up.

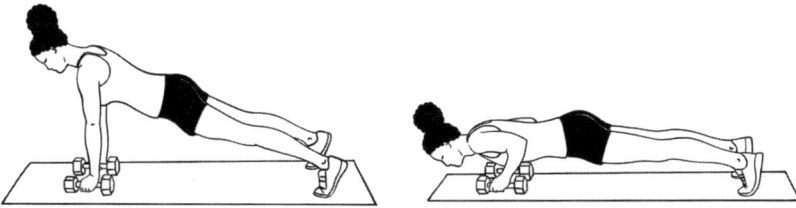

CORE FINISHER (4 minutes total)

Russian twists. (2 minutes) Grab just one heavy dumbbell and hold it on one side with both hands. Sit down on the floor, lean back, then lift and twist the dumbbell from side to side, tapping the floor near the hip. This is a spicy core workout but it is also great for your hip flexors and your lower back.

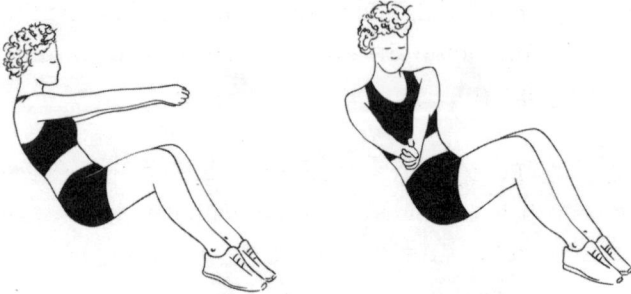

Mountain climbers. (2 minutes) Start in a high plank with your hands directly under your shoulders and your body in a straight line. Drive your right knee up towards your chest then return it, quickly switching legs so that your left knee comes forward as your right knee goes back. Keep alternating so that you're running horizontally. This is a long time, so it's okay to slow down or bring your knees down for rest whenever you need it! (See page 49.)

COOL DOWN (2 minutes)

Forward fold. Lower yourself down and let your upper body fold over your legs towards your feet. Let your head and neck hang loose.

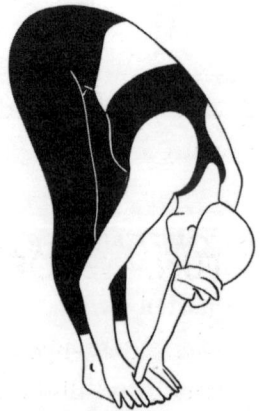

Cross-body shoulder stretch. Pull one hand across your body with the other hand, then switch over to the other side. (See page 108.)

Cat cow. On your hands and knees, arch your back and then curve it in again. (You should already know how to do this from the yoga section on page 81.)

Side stretch. Reach your arms up and grab your wrist with one hand. Stretch to the side of the hand that is holding on. Then switch to the other side.

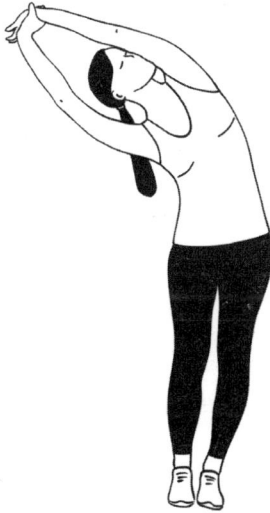

Give yourself a little round of applause for completing the workout. Champion!

FUN: THE FOR-THE-RECORD CHALLENGE

In this challenge, the word 'record' has a double meaning (I know, smart!). It's all about breaking your own records and tracking your own progress, but it *also* involves hitting 'record' on your phone and filming yourself.

Don't panic! These videos don't need to go anywhere other than your camera roll (unless you want them to). This is more about having a visual record of the progress you're making, giving yourself real-time feedback and allowing you to track improvements over time. Not only will you see your weight bands increasing, you'll also notice your form improving, your stamina cranking up a gear and your body changing. By rewatching these videos, you gain self-awareness of your form and where you need to improve. Think of it like a visual diary – not of before-and-after pics, but of you actually *doing the damn thing*.

Here's how it's gonna work.

Choose your moves. Pick a few exercises that you'd like to improve on. I'd suggest that these are exercises where you use free weights, so you can more easily see those bad-boys getting chunkier and chunkier. But it's truly up to you. Here are some examples of moves to choose:

Sumo squats: A wide-legged squat holding either a heavy dumbbell at your chest or a kettlebell hanging between your legs.

Bicep curls: You've done these a few times already now; holding dumbbells in each hand and activating your biceps to bring them up towards your chest.

Overhead press: Push those dumbbells up into the sky.

V-ups: This is a great exercise for activating those six-pack muscles. Lying flat on your mat, holding a dumbbell, extend your arms straight overhead (biceps by your ears), with your knees together and legs straight, toes pointed. Then exhale to simultaneously lift your legs and upper body off the ground into a v-shape, reaching the dumbbell towards your legs. Hold, then lower with control.

Push-ups: Starting on your knees and then progressing to a full push-up, this can be a really good one to assess strength and progress – even without added weights.

Record yourself. Set up your camera from a good angle to see yourself doing your move. Start recording when you're not feeling super confident with the move and your weights are light as hell. That's the whole point, friend – so you can see your progress right from a beginner. Then, you're going to want to record yourself at this exact same angle each week, performing the same amount of reps. Do this every week for as long as you like. It could take a few months before you reach the point where you think, 'wow, how the hell did I improve *that* much?!' Remember: if you never stop, you never fail.

OPTIONAL: You can keep the vids soundless or you can narrate them a little, saying how you felt doing the move or giving a thumbs-up to the camera. Your call.

Stitch the vids together. You can either keep adding to an extended video as you go along, or you can stitch it all together once you feel you have reached a place you're proud of. This is easily done on Instagram reels, TikTok or other good video-editing apps. You don't need to share it publicly if you don't want to – simply save the video in your drafts so that *you* get to see how well you have improved. And you never know, watching that progress could make you feel like you *do* want to celebrate publicly. If that's the case, go for it! Starting something that feels hard and then watching yourself become more and more comfortable, energised and strong is something to shout about from the rooftops, if you ask me. I'd love to see your compilations.

Remember, the only records you need to count are your own.

GET THE GANG INVOLVED

FOCUS: BUDDY UP

There ain't nothin' like team spirit, amirite? Growing up on sports teams, I have always loved the sense of camaraderie you have when you're working towards a common goal alongside other people. There's no 'I' in team, and you need to think beyond just yourself and your own needs. You have their backs, they have yours, and you're inspired to work harder because you don't want to let the team down. There's something powerful about working together – it makes you feel like you're never on your own, and everyone has an important role to play.

But you don't need a sports team to feel this sense of togetherness. You can find buddies to enhance your fitness journey. People who inspire you, motivate you and give you a safe space to mess up and pick yourself back up again. In the same way it benefits you to have a coach or personal trainer holding you accountable, it'll also make a huge difference if you have loved ones by your side, supporting you and cheering you on along the way. We are social creatures, after all. No one said you needed to go it alone.

Look, I know the idea of working out with other people can be intimidating – especially if you're only just starting out and everyone around you seems to be running like Mo Farah. You might assume that you'll feel embarrassed or deflated, so it's easier to stick to solo movement. Or you might have the opposite problem – it could be hard to find other people who are passionate about fitness in the same way, so you're forced to ride solo purely out of necessity.

However, I think it's really worth finding someone – even if it's just one person – to go on this journey with you (even occasionally). And you could even find that person in an unexpected place.

I gotta say, I never imagined that my favourite workout buddy would be my old mum. But the Covid-19 pandemic did weird things to all of us, didn't it? Moving back in with her after years of travelling the world, I felt extremely restless and upset that I couldn't train. The gym was my happy place, honestly, and when they all closed their doors, I felt pretty lost and knew my mental health would suffer if I didn't find a way around it. Mum agreed to help me convert a corner of the garage into a gym so I could keep on top of my fitness while we still didn't have a bleeding clue when we'd be free to live normally again.

As I've mentioned before, Mum has always been active, but with so many other things going on in her life (working full-time, raising kids), fitness had generally been on the backburner. During lockdown, with little else to do, she started taking an interest in what I was up to in that gym, and she asked me to help her learn the ropes with strength-training. Again, because I had *literally nothing else to do*, I agreed (and also because she birthed me, so I can't exactly say 'no' to the woman, can I?). I really didn't expect that training with my mum would be just as beneficial for me as it was for her.

First of all, it was a lovely opportunity for us to bond and connect, especially during a time when connection felt hard to come by. I've always had a great relationship with ol' Mum, but it got even stronger as we laughed when she stumbled, or when I congratulated her and told her I was proud of her when she moved up a weight bracket. When the weather was nice, we started heading out for runs together. Up until then, I had only known one gear: training for matches and races, pushing myself as hard as possible. With Mum, I wanted to run alongside her, so I had to take a different approach; to slow down and enjoy the process. On the other side of the coin, Mum told me that she learned so much from our workouts. Now, she has all the tools to do them on her own, but it's still much more enjoyable for both of us when we do it together!

The content I post with Mum has always been my most popular, and I think there's a reason why it has resonated. Not just to show that you can absolutely get fit at any age, but also to show that you can be workout buddies with anyone – no matter the differences in your experience, age, personal goals or motivation. The important thing is that you have the right attitude. If you're a beginner, you can utilise the more-experienced person to inspire you and motivate you. And if you're the more advanced buddy, you can use this opportunity to slow down, enjoy the journey and get back to basics. Plus, you also get a kick out of helping someone achieve their full potential. I blimmin' love helping people and making them feel good about themselves, as that makes *me* feel good in return. It's a win-win for everyone involved.

If you're still unconvinced, I'm gonna break down really simply why it can be so helpful to work out with other people . . .

The sense of community. I'd define a community as a group of people with common interests, who are working towards a common goal. Whether you're attending a run-club or gym class, or just working out with a mate, this is exactly what you're doing. You feed off the group energy, which lifts you up. I think it's mega inspiring to look around you and realise that other people are also doing the best they can to become that healthier version of themselves. When we feel like we're part of something and we belong, it can feel like a safer and less-intimidating environment to strive towards good health.

Learning and inspiration. If someone is more experienced than you, it can be helpful to learn from them and feel inspired. You might have heard this saying: 'If you're the smartest person in the room, then you're in the wrong room.' Well, the same goes for fitness. Being 'better' than everyone around you can actually be detrimental, because how are you going to improve? When I played professional rugby, I really looked up to the more experienced members of the team. They supported me, and they set an example that I could follow. I also love working out with people who put me through my paces – as they make me strive to do better. And anyway, there's always something you can learn from someone else, whether they're more experienced or not – just like I learned heaps from my ol' mum. Perhaps it's their attitude, or the way they put in so much effort to push harder when they feel like giving up. Being around others = inspiration galore!

It becomes a social occasion. Oh, how I love to multi-task. Working out with my mates essentially kills two birds with one stone (don't worry, no *actual* birds are harmed – only metaphorical ones). I get to move my body, get those endorphins flowing and look jacked as well as hang out and have a catch-up with the people I love. The best part is, you can combine it with a coffee or even book in a G&T for afterwards, adding *another* benefit of that positive reinforcement we talked about in the last level. This entire book is about making exercise fun (in case ya hadn't noticed) and enjoying it with friends is such an easy way to do that. Job done!

They can hold you accountable. Yes sir, here's that accountability word again! Truly, you wouldn't cancel on your friends, would you? (At least I hope not.) So if you book a 9 a.m. class or run with your pal, you're much more likely to show up because you don't want to let them down. Not only that, once you're there, they can encourage you to keep going – being that external motivational voice that is *always* helpful.

Science says so. There has been plenty of research into the benefits of exercising with other people, whether that's with your friends and family, or a group setting like a class or run-club. One recent study found that social exercise improved people's wellbeing, because it enhanced the possibility for social connection.[1] That makes sense, given we know that loneliness can be as dangerous for you as smoking. Another study found that people were likely to lose more weight if they had others around them who were also motivated to lose weight.[2] Again, we vibe off other people's energy. If you don't trust me, trust the science.

Still, I know these benefits won't always take away the actual fear of putting this into practice. It can feel vulnerable to share your journey with others, so here are my top tips for buddying up in the right way – to really get the most out of all the benefits and enhance your workouts by a mile . . .

Be conscious about your circle. If you're afraid to exercise with someone because you're concerned that they might disparage you or put you down, that's probably not someone you want in your life, let alone someone to work out with. The right people will always encourage you and reassure you. If it's someone you really care about, and they care about you, it's probably more likely your critical voice making you believe that they'll judge you or make you feel bad. It's not *actually* the truth. Be discerning about the person you ask to join you; if

---

1   https://www.sciencedirect.com/science/article/pii/S0277953623008110?via%3Dihub
2   https://pmc.ncbi.nlm.nih.gov/articles/PMC3676749/

you surround yourself with good people (which I'm sure you already do), I promise it'll be more enjoyable than you think. The right person will help you to step outside your comfort zone and elevate your training to new heights. So just think carefully about who that person could be. I exercise with a lot of other people who prioritise the same things that I do. They value being healthy, but they're not too strict about it. They still love a beer in the pub after lifting some weights. Surround yourself with good people who share your values, and you'll feel all those uplifting wellness benefits.

HOW TO CHOOSE THE RIGHT WORKOUT BUDDY

It doesn't matter if they're more or less experienced, older or younger, man or woman, hairy or bald. Just make sure they tick all these boxes . . .

- They value health and fitness, just like you.

- They have your best interests at heart.

- They are kind and non-judgemental.

- You enjoy being around them.

- You admire them in some way – maybe it's their effort, how they prioritise and organise their life, or their resilience to push through challenges.

AND IF YOU DON'T THINK YOU KNOW ANYONE WHO TICKS ALL THESE BOXES . . .

You can find them! Joining a gym, fitness community or run-club is a great way to find like-minded people.

Book classes. In the same way you might pay a little more for a fun day out with your friends, it's a good idea to book something you wouldn't normally attend. Maybe it's aerial yoga where you hang from the ceiling like a bat, or even a hardcore HIIT sweat-sesh, or maybe a spin class with pumping music that feels like you're in a nightclub. Even if you go alone, these kinds of classes feel like an occasion – you can usually find them in fancier studios with nice changing rooms, making the whole experience feel like a treat. Plus, the energy in the room gives you that sense of togetherness.

Join a Parkrun. If you love running, you can find one of these in almost every town or city. It's basically a big communal run – usually not longer than 5k. Totally low-pressure and low-stakes, but you get the benefits of running with a pack, feeling like you're part of a community and being inspired by the people around you.

Get friends and fam involved. Just like I did with my mum, you can get your friends and family involved. For one, they love you unconditionally (I hope) and they're more likely to care about your best interests. Exercising with kids can be such a great way to set a good example about prioritising health and fitness at every stage of life. There's a family I always see in my local park on Saturday mornings – parents running, kids cycling alongside. I love that, because they're just having fun in the park on the weekend, but they're also all moving as a unit, and the kids are learning the value (and fun) of exercise.

Keep it fun and light. Cast your mind back to Level 1 and you'll remember that fitness isn't only about structured workouts and gym regimes, it's about moving your body in feelgood ways. When my partner and I go on holiday together, one of our favourite ways to spend a day is to find a beautiful view for a long hike (the hillier and sweatier the better). It's such a great way to see a new place, plus it is good for us, especially if we might not have access to a gym or our usual kit. The even-better part is finding somewhere afterwards for a drink and some food, then chilling for the rest of the day on the beach. We really feel like we've earned it. Name a better feeling!

FEAR: YOUR ONLY COMPETITION? YOU!

Anyone who has played a sport to a high level knows there's one quality you absolutely need in order to succeed – that's a competitive streak. Whether you're on a team or you're a solo ranger in athletics, you've got to be in it to win it. Do you think Dina Asher-Smith, Lewis Hamilton or David Beckham would've reached all their achievements if they hadn't had that burning desire to win? Sure, natural talent comes into it, but in order to win, you have to train hard, stay focused and keep your head in the game. You have to want it more than anyone else. That's how true champions are made.

'But Tom, I thought you said I shouldn't train like an athlete?' You're absolutely right. You don't need the same level of competitiveness as athletes. If you're reading this book, I'm assuming you're not a full-time athlete – you have your own career, responsibilities and priorities. You're not looking at competing in the Olympics, you're just trying to have a healthier lifestyle. So you don't need to emulate an athlete in all respects. However, as you progress through your fitness journey and become much more comfortable and consistent with the rhythms of your exercise routine, you may want to step it up a notch. You may want to push yourself and see what you're really made of. You might want to get *in it to win it*, just to see if you can.

This is absolutely optional. If you never want to sign up for a challenge or join a race ever in your life, then you do you! However,

I want to make the case for setting yourself a scary goal. Signing up for something can give you the push you need to step into the most resilient, determined, motivated version of yourself. It can add a little extra reason onto your deeper 'why', fuelling you to keep going and push yourself to the edge. It's a way of holding yourself accountable and making sure you're staying on track, because you're working towards something real and tangible. And it teaches you, in real time, to get comfortable with failure, because sometimes you *won't* perform to the best of your abilities, or achieve your goal, and *that's okay,* because everyone loves a comeback story.

Essentially, a little competition can be a good way to test all of your deep-rooted fears surrounding fitness. If you think you're ready, or you want a little push, signing up for something could be the difference between scraping by and unlocking your true potential. To infinity, and beyond!

I know I'm biased. I've already told you that I got pretty obsessed with competing in races and challenges after my rugby career ended. That competitive streak needed somewhere to go, so I channelled it into various challenges – from marathons to triathlons – because I loved having that fire in my belly. I loved the nervous feeling I'd get before each competition, as it exposed a sort of vulnerability in me that I leaned into and enjoyed. It's the ultimate mindset test. You have to dig really deep to push through a challenge. You have to find resilience that you're not even sure exists (until you find it). This isn't just a standard gym sesh – you're under pressure, and sometimes that can be good for the soul. I gotta say, race day is a rush and that euphoric feeling you get after crossing the finish line is second to none.

And, yes, I know what you're thinking: *'But Tom, that didn't exactly end well, did it? You screwed up your spine!'* While that's absolutely true, I want to make clear that this was more to do with my own obsession and doing too much all at once, believing I was invincible. Had I chosen just one competition at a time, and prioritised my recovery, it would've been a different story. So I still recommend setting yourself these goals but being really realistic about where you're at in your journey, and what your body can handle. If you're a complete beginner at running you're probably not going to be smashing out a half marathon any time soon, but you could absolutely sign up for a 5k, or even a 10k (if you give yourself a date far enough into the future to build your training gradually). Challenges don't have to be absolutely huge – no one is expecting you to complete an ultra marathon straight off the bat (see page 159) – it's more about starting with something that feels hard *to you*. Not to anyone else.

You see, the set-up of competitions and challenges might seem like you're competing against other people. And, yes, professional athletes will absolutely view it that way. However, the vast majority of people competing in events are only competing with one person – and that's themselves. I've said it before and I'll say it again, your fitness journey is a game of you versus you. Even when you're in a group event environment, that point still stands. There might be other people cycling next to you as you're furiously pushing your pedals, but they don't matter in the slightest. What matters is that *you* are pushing yourself, and you are becoming even 1 per cent stronger than you were yesterday – whether that's physically or emotionally. What matters is that *you* reach that finish line feeling mega proud of everything you have achieved and all the hurdles you overcame to get there.

Plus, you get that community feel of travelling in a pack. You don't need to be competing with the people around you. You don't need to be going faster than them, working harder than them, showing off your muscles more than them. You can just absorb the energy of people around you – from all different backgrounds, with their own stories of why they're there – and let that sense of togetherness fill your cup right up.

One client, Maria*, told me when we first met that she absolutely hated running, and she would never, ever run a marathon. I'm always taken aback when people say things like this. The word 'never' simply doesn't exist in my vocabulary. Who are we to say something so definitive? We all change and grow and expand, you simply can't know what your future holds, what might capture your heart and what you're capable of.

Anyway, Maria started small on her journey. She began with strength-training and very short runs, just to get her into the groove. It turned out she actually quite liked running, and she told me she started to enjoy the unique combination of peace and challenge that it brought her. Still, she had no intention of competing in any race and instead stuck to 'easy-peasy' 2–5k runs around her local park.

And then the unthinkable happened. Her husband was diagnosed with stage 4 cancer and deteriorated quickly. Suddenly, Maria's running took on a new purpose; it helped her to process, to come to terms with the possibility of losing the love of her life. It also motivated her to set a goal. In a bid to raise money for the cancer charity that was making a huge difference in her husband's life, she set herself the challenge of running a half marathon. Raising money for this charity that meant so much to her added more meaning to her runs, helping her push through the pain, and taking on each new step in her training with a fire in her belly. I always say that the training is the real race – that's the tough part, where you really have to dig deep; the race itself is really just a victory lap and a celebration. This is where you get to see all that hard work pay off.

Maria told me that crossing the finish line of her half marathon was euphoric. Not only because she had achieved something she never thought she would, but because she had raised over £1,000 for her chosen charity. And her husband was there, cheering her on.

After he passed away, she didn't want to give up. She wanted to ensure his legacy lived on. Now she has run three marathons in different cities around the world and raised thousands of pounds for charity. Of course, you don't need a tragic incident to inspire you to take on a challenge (and I really hope you don't experience one!), but Maria's story is a reminder of a few things. Firstly, never say 'never', because life comes at you fast and your priorities and motivations can change. And, secondly, remember that fitness challenges can provide an incredible sense of purpose. Maria is a bloody inspiration, and she proves that we all have that fire inside us. It's up to us if we want to answer the call.

Life is tough, but you are tougher.

Competitions you could try

You absolutely do not need to throw yourself into a marathon to feel the benefits and camaraderie of joining a competition or race. It's all about starting small, seeing how it feels and then taking on more and more if you're getting something out of it. Here are some comps you could try, starting from total beginner up to advanced athlete.

Metric classes

This could barely be classified as a race, but it's a good way to dip your feet into fitness with a competitive edge. Many fitness classes include some kind of leaderboard or way of tracking your metrics, even if that's just a light that pops up on your spin-bike to show how much effort you're putting in. Some people hate this and prefer to stay in their own bubble during their workouts, but seeing your name up on a leaderboard and pushing to get it higher and higher can help you improve week on week. Lots of my clients have found this surprisingly motivating. You probably won't know any of the other people you're competing against – it's all about how much *you're* improving.

Charity fun runs

If you want a low-pressure race to sign up to, charity fun runs pop up anywhere and everywhere. With these, you raise money for a specific cause while running a fairly short distance (often 5k, but they can be even shorter). There's always a really fun, lively atmosphere; they are completely low pressure, but a great way to see if you enjoy that kind of environment.

Cycling sportives

If you're not a runner but you love being on your bike and still want that challenge, a sportive could be the perfect thing for you. These are essentially organised, long-distance bike rides that often involve cycling between cities or towns along certain routes. Once again, you're not competing directly against the other riders, but you are timing yourself, so it's all about your personal achievement (but remember – personal bests are also about feelings, rather than numbers!). Lots of sportives include different route options, ranging from beginner-friendly to more advanced, meaning they're super inclusive.

Obstacle course races

These are fun competitions if you want to have a good day out with your mates and get a little dirty (oo-er). The most popular ones in the UK include Tough Mudder and Spartan Sprint – you complete 5–10k worth of challenges, dealing with mud, ropes and walls. They're great for building teamwork, and if you love being a big kid.

Indoor fitness races

A bit like obstacle courses but with a stricter fitness focus, competitions like CrossFit and HYROX are massively popular these days. Both use team or pair formats (meaning it's a great way to get the gang involved, working towards a common goal). They involve a mix of different kinds of strength and cardio exercises, with CrossFit also involving extra Olympic-style challenges. Definitely more advanced, but incredible if you love a challenge and get a buzz from the competition environment.

Triathlons/marathons

Now, *this* is where I really come alive! These are proper long-distance races that will challenge you in every way – mind, body and soul. Triathlons often include a 750m swim, 20k bike and 5k run, while marathons see strong-minded legends run for 26.2 miles. Both require a lot of training to complete the goal, which, as I said before, is often the hardest part. Completing a challenge like this is truly no better feeling.

Ultra marathons/Ironman/Extreme challenges

This might seem completely out of your ballpark right now, but who knows, maybe one day you'll sign up for an ultra marathon, which is essentially anything longer than a marathon (and sometimes races span about 250k in five days. Truly wild). Or you could try an Ironman – a super-long triathlon which involves a 3.8k swim, 180k bike ride and a marathon run. Then there are also trail marathons (where you're going uphill on rocky terrain), plus there are tons of cool races around the world that see people take on desert and snow conditions. Pretty intense, if you ask me, and I think you'd have to be a bit of a sucker for punishment, but still, it's possible!

Keeping competition healthy

The trick about getting involved with events and competitions is that it should always *feel good*. That doesn't mean it won't be tough. By golly, it'll be tough. But it'll be tough in a good way. The kind of tough that makes you feel alive. The kind of tough that makes you feel proud. The kind of tough that makes you feel unstoppable. That's the kind of tough that'll fill you to the brim with happy chemicals and keep you coming back for more.

But remember, competitions aren't about comparison. Yes, you're doing them alongside other people, but it doesn't matter what those other people are doing. You can soak in their presence, the camaraderie and community without measuring yourself against them. When one of my clients crossed the finish line of a marathon with a time of 5 hours 45 minutes, I couldn't have been prouder of him – and he couldn't have been prouder of himself. We all have our own times, distances and goals that we're working towards, and those targets are no less or more worthy than anyone else's. We're all on our own fitness adventures, which is absolutely bloody beautiful.

Once again, I want to remind you that you don't ever need to sign up for a race or event if you don't want to. If you'd prefer to keep your exercise routine free from pressure, then I absolutely commend you for that. What I want to show you, though, is that if you wanted to sign up for something, you absolutely could. You have the capability, the resilience and the strength to try. You don't need to be the best. You don't need to win. Just showing up is the most important part. So if you want to give something a go, just imagine I'm there, cheering you on from the sidelines.

FITNESS: LET'S GET SWEATY

If you've been doing the workouts so far, you shouldn't be any stranger to getting sweaty. Cardio exercise is a great way to get your heart pumping fresh blood around your body, and lifting heavy weights can also help you work up a sweat. But now it's time to push your body to the limits and test out some High Intensity Interval Training (HIIT).

What is HIIT?

This is a workout structure where you alternate between short bursts of intense exercise, followed by brief recovery periods. These are the kinds of workouts that can really get your heart pumping, making your breathing shallower and making you sweat profusely. You may be thinking: *'Sounds painful, why would I want to do that?'* Well, there are tons of benefits of HIIT. Not only is it time-efficient, it improves oxygen consumption, reduces heart rate and improves blood pressure – all of which help with shedding weight and gaining muscle. When you work out in intense bursts you also burn more calories both during and after exercise, so even when you're resting, you're burning.[3]

However, it's important to note that HIIT is best done in moderation. HIIT puts your body under stress, and while we know that this can be a good thing if you want to see a transformation, you also shouldn't put your body under *too* much stress. Too much HIIT could lead to overtraining injuries, plus being in a calorie deficit could also negatively impact your hormones. So do these kinds of workouts sparingly – once or twice a week is enough.

3   https://pmc.ncbi.nlm.nih.gov/articles/PMC8294064/

HIIT workouts can include so many different elements – they almost always include some element of cardio, whether that's jumping, running or cycling sprints, and many also include strength-training elements to keep things spicy.

In this HIIT workout you can do the entire thing at home, without any equipment. You don't need to run or cycle, but the jumping element of these moves adds the cardio factor.

Note: Keep a towel handy. You're gonna need it. And remember to stay hydrated, drinking sips of water in breaks between movements. This will help you recover all that moisture you lose through sweat!

YOUR 30-MINUTE HOME SWEAT FEST

WARM-UP (5 minutes)

Spend about a minute on each of the following moves (or you can extend this part to really warm yourself up – totally up to you!).

Shoulder rolls and arm circles. Roll those shoulders back and forth and make circles with your arms, one way then another. This should feel really good and will loosen up those limbs!

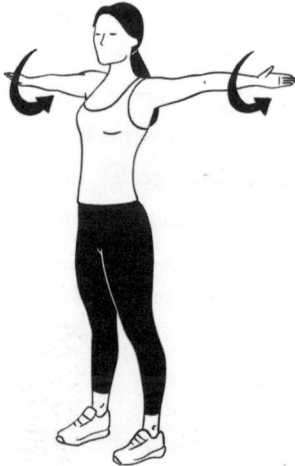

World's greatest stretch. We've done this before – simply step one foot forward into a low lunge, with your back knee on the floor. Lift the opposite arm high to the sky, then return to standing and repeat on the other side. (See page 107.)

Downward dog. From a plank position, lift your hips and bum up to the sky, keeping your back as straight as possible. Take your dog for a walk (moving your feet back and forth and even doing some ankle circles). Great for waking up the whole body. (See page 82.)

Jog in place. Now you're really warming up – simply jog on the spot, lifting your knees high.

Bodyweight squats. Lower down into slow, controlled squats to warm up the glutes and knees. (See page 139.)

MAIN 20-MIN HIIT CIRCUIT (20 minutes)

Here you have 9 different moves – complete each one for 40 seconds, with a 20-second rest in between. Once you've completed a round, take a 1-minute break, then repeat all 9 moves and take a 1-minute break before starting the cool down.

(If you're just getting started, you might want to try just one round for a shorter workout.)

Star jumps/Jumping jacks. You might remember doing these in school, but trust me, they really get your heart thumping. Start standing up tall, feet together, with your arms by your sides. Jump your feet out wide while

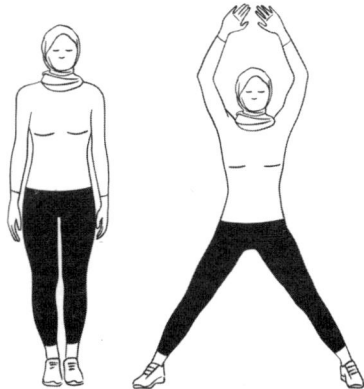

swinging your arms out into a star shape (or overhead). Jump your feet back together, bringing your arms back to your sides. Keep going as quickly as you can for the full 40 seconds.

Squat jumps. Standing with your feet hip-width apart, lower into a squat, putting your weight into your heels, hips back, chest up. To come out of it, explosively jump up, swinging your arms up overhead. Land softly, before immediately lowering back into the squat.

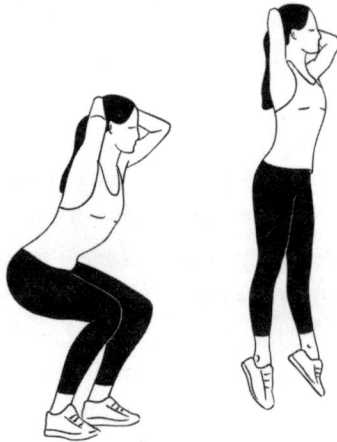

Curtsy lunges. Stand tall with your feet hip-width apart. Step your right foot back, behind your left leg at an angle, so it looks like a curtsy. Bend both knees to lower down, with your front knee over your ankle and your back knee pointing towards the floor. Push through your front heel to return to standing, then repeat on the other side. The faster you do these, the sweatier you'll get, but slower and controlled means a more noticeable burn.

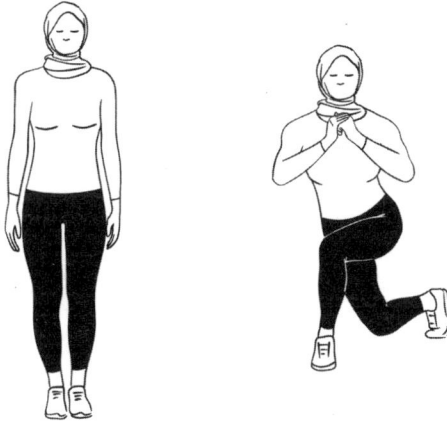

Burpees. This dreaded move is key in any HIIT routine. Stand tall with your feet shoulder-width apart. Squat down and place your hands on the floor. Then jump or step your feet back into a high plank. From there, do a push-up – either a full one or with your knees down. Jump up to step your feet back towards your hands, then explosively jump up, reaching your arms above your head. Move at a steady pace and prioritise quality of movement over speed

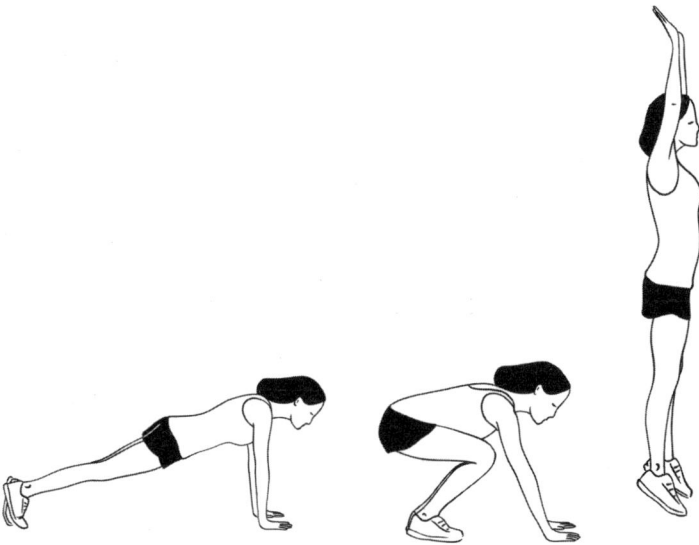

Plank shoulder taps. From a high-plank position – hands under shoulders, body in a straight line, with feet slightly wider than hip-width apart – lift your right hand to tap your left shoulder. Return your hand to the floor, then lift your left hand to tap your right shoulder. Engage your core to keep your hips from swaying. Increase the speed if you can, remaining as stable as possible in your hips. (See page 47.)

Mountain climbers. Also starting in a high-plank position, drive your right knee in towards your chest. Quickly switch, driving your left knee in, as you extend your right knee back. Keep alternating in a quick 'running' motion. (See page 49.)

Push-ups. As many as you can do – slow and controlled, or faster for more of a sweat. From a high plank, bend your elbows to lower your chest towards the floor, keeping them at a 45-degree angle to your torso. Press through your palms to push up. Modify and make things a bit easier by putting your knees down.

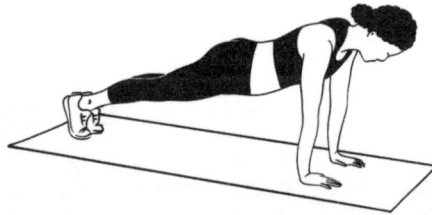

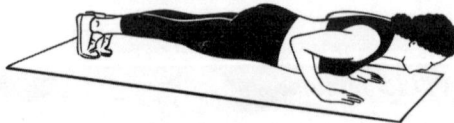

Ab crunches. Lie on your back, with your knees bent and feet flat on the floor. With your hands behind your head and elbows wide, engage your abs to lift your shoulders and upper back off the floor, then lower down with control. Make sure you're not pulling your neck – you should be lifting up using your abs.

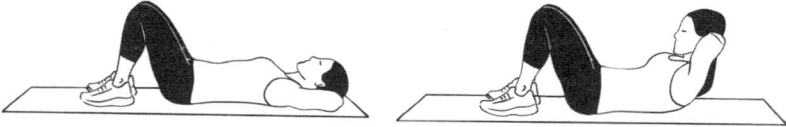

Bicycle crunches. Lie on your back, with your knees bent and hands behind your head, supporting your neck. Lift your shoulders off the floor and bring your right elbow towards your left knee as you extend your right leg out straight. Then switch sides – left elbow to right knee, left leg outstretched. Continue in a pedalling motion – a bit like riding a bike. Make sure you stay controlled, twisting from your torso and keeping your core engaged. The faster you go, the sweatier it'll be, but make sure you don't sacrifice that form.

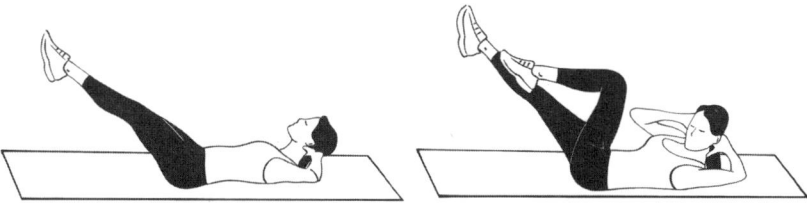

COOL-DOWN (5 minutes)

You've probably generated quite a significant amount of heat, so you're gonna enjoy this cool-down! Spend about a minute on each move – or even longer if it feels good.

Quad stretch. Stand tall and grab your right ankle with your right hand, pulling your heel towards your glutes behind you. Keep your knees close together and push your hips forward just a little. This should feel great after all those jumps, squats and lunges.

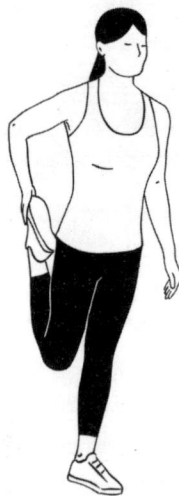

Forward fold. Hinge at the hips to let your upper body hang heavy towards the floor. It's totally fine to have a slight bend in your knees. (See page 142.)

Cat cow. This is great for your spine but also for just focusing on your breathing and calming down your body. From all fours, drop your belly and lift your head while inhaling for cow, then round your back and tuck your chin in while exhaling for cat. (See page 82.)

Figure-four stretch. While lying on your back, lift your legs into the air and cross the right ankle over your left thigh to look like a '4' shape. Pull your left leg in towards you, for a deep stretch in your hip and glute. Then switch sides.

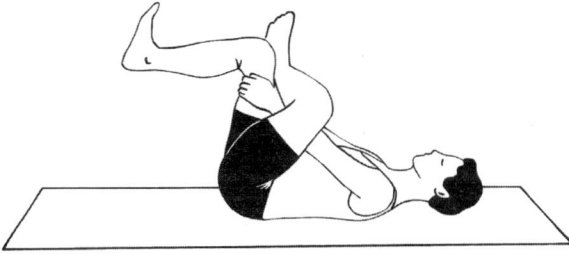

Child's pose. Now it's time to let it all hang out. Kneel on the floor, with your big toes touching and your knees wide. Sit your hips back towards your heels, reach your arms forward and melt your forehead down to the floor. Breathe deeply and say to yourself, 'I'm a bloody legend.'

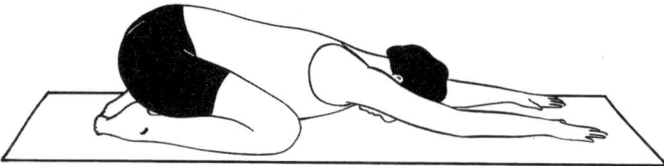

FUN: SPORTS DAY FOR GROWN-UPS

Sports day games aren't just for kids, and they aren't just for fun either. Organising your very own sports day is a great way to get the gang involved with movement and getting fit. Plus, many of your favourite playground games are actually *genuinely* good for working towards your fitness goals – they're ideal forms of cardio, working various different muscle groups as well as challenging your mobility and balance. Except you won't really feel like you're working out, because you'll be busy having a laugh with your mates and racing for that gold prize. Talk about a win-win!

This works best if you go to a park or have a big garden. (I'd recommend not doing these games inside, for safety reasons. And your mum/other half may want to kill you. Learn from my mistakes.)

Here's how it'll work . . .

Create your teams. It's totally up to you how you designate teams – you could have pairs, triples or even bigger groups depending on how many people you have involved. Each team creates their own competitive name. The sillier the better.

Draw up a scoreboard. This could be a chalk-board, a whiteboard, a giant piece of paper, or even a note on your phone if you're keeping things under a strict budget. After each game, note the team winner down on the board, so you can keep track – and keep that competitive spirit going through each game.

Choose your prizes. It's not about winning, it's about taking part. Still, a little trophy or medal never hurt nobody. You could buy (or make) some gold, silver and bronze medals, but feel free to get more creative than that. You could also have a prize for 'best team player' or 'funniest fall'. (Remember, it's all in jest – no need to take things too seriously!)

Play your games! There are so many sports day games you can choose from, and you can do as many or as few as you like. Here are some of my favourites, plus why they *actually* count as a workout.

Egg and spoon race. Pretty much the most classic sports day race – the goal is to reach the finish line first with your egg (carried balanced on a spoon) still intact. Not only does this test your speed, it also tests your stability and balance. If you've been working hard at Pilates, you'll see it pay off here!

Sack race. Another childhood classic. Each person stands in a big sack (or pillowcase) and hops to the finish line. You'll be working your calves, glutes and quads while you get pretty out of breath and build your cardio fitness, too.

Tug of war. Two teams pull on the opposite ends of a sturdy rope, and the first team to drag someone from the other team across the centre line wins. You'll notice if your upper body strength work has started paying off here – this will really test your upper back and triceps, but it'll also challenge your grip strength and legs, as you'll want to stay as sturdy as possible to avoid getting dragged over the line!

Obstacle course. You can set this up however you like – and really feel free to get creative. Set up hoops for jumping into, tunnels for crawling through, obstacles to jump over – you could even add in a drinking game or challenge or two. Depending on what you implement, this can be a total-body workout, and it also exercises the mind as you need to think about what you're doing next!

Wheelbarrow race. In pairs, one person becomes a human wheelbarrow by walking on their hands while their partner holds their ankles. This is a workout for everyone involved – if you're on your hands, you'll be training your shoulders, core, arms and chest. And if you're the one pushing the wheelbarrow, you'll feel it in your legs and your grip.

Skipping race. Using a skipping rope is an incredible form of cardio, while also testing your rhythm and coordination. Getting to the finish line quickly using a skipping rope is surprisingly tricky.

Hula-hoop tournament. Keep the hula-hoop whizzing around your waist – last one to drop theirs wins! Hula-hooping is another childhood toy that works as a form of cardio, while also strengthening your core, balance and coordination.

Whichever games you choose, be sure to give 'em your all, have fun with your pals and make core memories. That's what life (and fitness) is all about.

IT'S A LIFESTYLE, BABY

FOCUS: HARNESS THE GOOD STUFF

So far, we have talked a lot about how fitness will benefit your health – you'll improve muscle tone, lose weight and boost your energy levels. We've also covered some of the great mental health benefits – exercise releases 'happy chemicals' like endorphins that flood our bodies and make us feel amazing. But if you can cast your mind back to the introduction (yep, there have been a *lot* of pages between then and now!), you might remember the promise I made to you: that a fitness lifestyle would help improve every area of your life – your mind, your body *and* your soul. And now I want to explain how that *really* happens.

I want to show you how exercise can enhance your relationships, your career, your hobbies and your everyday wellbeing. It's not just about the time you spend in the gym, lifting the weights or pounding the pavements, it's about *everything* you learn about yourself from these moments. It's about all the incredible things you gain – the things that last even when you've showered off all the sweat and you're getting on with your day. We've hinted at some of these themes the whole way through this book, but now's the time to really appreciate just how bloody fantastic fitness can be for your overall life. It's a game-changer, I'm tellin' ya.

First of all, I want you to reflect on your own life since you started working through this book and building up your fitness. Have you noticed any changes beyond just your workout routine and your body shape? Have you noticed any changes in your relationships, your career, your general lifestyle? You might have experienced some positive developments but assumed they were completely separate to your newfound love of exercise. And that could be true. But I'd also guarantee that exercise played a role – whether directly or more subtly.

Don't believe me? Here are some of the main ways in which fitness can improve your life overall. I've seen them happen (with my own eyes) to loved ones and clients, again and again.

Fitness is a snowball

When you start implementing a structured exercise routine, you might notice that it becomes easier to stick to other healthy habits. This is because you're already in the flow of looking after yourself and prioritising your health, so, naturally, it makes you want to do *more*. One study found that participants who stuck to an exercise regime were more likely to eat healthily.[1] It's hard to know exactly why this happens, but I think that good health fuels more good health. Once you start, you want to keep going.

Then there's the fact that exercising can actually help you to sleep better, which we know is a massive factor in feeling great all day long (we'll cover sleep in the next Fear section, which is all about recovery). Waking up earlier to exercise may force you to get outside in the mornings, which helps you to set your body clock

1   https://www.nature.com/articles/s41366-018-0299-3

(also known as your 'circadian rhythm'), which can also help you sleep better at night.

You may also find that when you're exercising your health suddenly becomes a *priority*. You look forward to your Saturday morning run-club, so overdoing it on the beers on a Friday night may not be so appealing anymore. (Running on a hangover is very possible . . . just not very enjoyable.) You might find that your self-control increases, so you reduce the booze, or smoking, or whatever other vices you have without even noticing; subconsciously cutting down as your priorities begin to shift. It's really just like a snowball, and once you get your fitness snowball rolling, before you know it, you're healthier than you ever thought possible.

This exact phenomenon happened to one of my clients, Dave*. When Dave came to me, he wanted to get fit, but that wasn't the only thing that needed to change in his life. As a freelancer, he had fallen into the habit of waking up late, then working late and ordering endless takeaways (his favourites were pizza and Chinese!). And given he wouldn't eat his dinner until 9.30 p.m., he'd stay up even later, so he'd need to have that lie-in . . . and the whole cycle made it impossible to implement healthy change.

When he came to me, I knew he needed a total routine overhaul. So, I told him to start waking up just one hour earlier (10.30 a.m instead of 11.30 a.m.) to fit in his workout. Then, we worked on some easy, healthy meal-prep so that he didn't feel the need to order takeaways while he was deep in focus-mode at his desk – he could simply reheat and tuck into something he'd already made. This felt like a big challenge at first, as waking up to work out and meal-prepping were not part of Dave's repertoire. But if you never make changes, you're never going to change.

What I love about Dave is that he put his trust in me, he did the prep, he woke up earlier – even though for the first couple of weeks it was an almighty struggle. He really relied on my accountability at this point. But over time it got easier and easier and, naturally, his whole routine shifted. He woke up earlier, exercised, and started tackling his workload before lunchtime. Then he worked through the afternoon before eating a healthy meal-prep dinner and even having some extra time for resting and socialising – catching up with friends, prioritising his hobbies – which had fallen by the wayside before. He could get to sleep earlier, which meant he didn't have any problems waking up earlier the next day. You see, your mornings affect your afternoons, your evenings and your nighttimes, which then affect your mornings. Your habits will either hurt or help your other habits. You can choose which route you'd prefer to go down.

The whole thing snowballed and eventually his days looked nothing like how they had just a few months earlier. Dave told me that life didn't feel like such a strain anymore. He no longer felt exhausted and sluggish. His motivation increased tenfold. He even started dating, and he met someone special. His fitness journey is just one example of the ultimate snowball. As soon as he changed one thing, everything else began to fall into place.

Fitness builds resilience

Throughout this book I've already told several stories about my clients' incredible resilience – their ability to push through challenges and persevere. They are genuinely amazing, and they inspire me every day! But it's not just that these people are particularly special. Of course, we're all special, but what I mean by that is *anyone* can build resilience through the very nature of exercising. The whole process of fitness is, in itself, about doing really hard stuff and making it out the other side. That is the definition of resilience. And if you don't feel like you're a particularly resilient person, exercise can bring it out of you. It's one of the biggest transferable skills you learn when you start to get fit.

Exercising is tough, and so is life. I've already spoken about how my mum's fitness journey allowed her to overcome being knocked off her bike and the shoulder injury she received. She's not the only one. My client, Timmy*, was made redundant a couple of months after we started working together. Over those first eight weeks, he had lifted weights for the first time and run his first 5k, after previously believing he'd be totally 'useless' (his words). Those improvements had taught him something incredibly valuable: he wasn't useless, not even a little bit. He could conquer difficult challenges. He could make it through.

Rather than being knocked down by his redundancy, his brain shifted gears. He thought: 'How can I get through this? How can I turn this experience into something positive?' He realised that he hadn't really loved his job for a long time (in fact, he'd probably *never* loved his job). It was a soulless office role where he felt like he was a cog in a machine – a fact which, in the face of redundancy, only became more real. He thought he would rather do something where he could make a difference, so he decided to retrain as a teacher. The training was tough – starting again in your late-thirties is no mean feat! But now he's doing what he does best – inspiring others – all while maintaining his exercise routine most mornings before school. What a legend.

When you lift a heavier weight, when you get through a long workout in one piece, when you tackle a move you never thought possible, you are teaching yourself valuable skills that you can apply in your everyday life. You teach yourself that 'hard' doesn't mean 'impossible'. You understand that 'tough' doesn't mean giving up. You gain evidence that difficult things can be overcome. And not just overcome but *turned into something bloody fantastic.* When the going gets tough, *you* get even tougher.

Fitness improves self-love

'Love yourself' might feel like an unrealistic thing to strive towards. But, to me, self-love is all about having a base level of compassion and respect for yourself. It's about having confidence, and knowing that you are still worthy of love, even if you're imperfect or mess up. And I believe that fitness is one of the best ways to build this kind of self-love.

This happens in several different ways. First of all, you draw on that lesson of resilience we just spoke about. Knowing that you *are* bloody capable, well, that's a massive confidence-builder. Self-love grows when you can look back at your achievements and think: 'Yep, I did that. I'm proud of myself. And I can do even *more*, just like that.'

Secondly, fitness can change the way you look – and in doing so, the way you feel about yourself and the way you carry yourself. In Level 2, we spoke about how aesthetics aren't everything – and I absolutely stand by that. Still, the better you *feel* about your appearance, the easier you will find it to show up as your best self. This definitely happened for my client, Hannah*, who lost 2 stone while we worked together. Before that, her confidence had been on the floor, which affected everything from her dating life to her career. She didn't put her hand up in meetings, and she tended to wear black, baggy clothes. She allowed herself to fade into the background because she preferred to hide herself.

But once she started losing weight, she began to view herself differently. She started buying new clothes in bright colours that made her feel amazing. As a result, she began to walk taller, holding her head high. She gained the confidence to speak up, and even decided that she wanted to apply for a promotion. She messaged me just after her interview with a quick snap in the mirror, saying: 'I felt so good about myself in that interview – I think I've smashed it!' And guess what? She did!

As I've said before, appearance definitely isn't everything, but it is a piece of the confidence puzzle. If you feel good in your own skin you'll shift the energy you put out into the world. You feel more comfortable getting out there and saying, 'This. Is. Me.'

I could go on and on about how fitness improves self-love. It's in the sense of reward you get after each session. It's in the pride you feel for waking up early, for making yourself a priority. It grows and grows, so subtly that you might not even notice it at first. Sometimes my clients need to be told that they are absolutely awesome before they start believing it themselves. Then when they do believe it, it becomes their default setting. It's one of my favourite things to witness.

Fitness teaches you to show up

Every time you put on your leggings and get your mat out in your living room. Every time you check into the gym. Every time you book onto a gym class (and actually follow through). All of these moments when you show up, you're gaining a valuable lesson. You're learning to show up for yourself, yes, but you're also learning to show up *in general* for whatever is important in your life. You're learning to be reliable and dependable. That's another ultimate transferable skill you get from exercising.

When I first met my client, Fred*, his marriage was on the rocks. That's not why he came to me, though. Obviously I am not a couples' therapist, but his wife thought it might be a good idea. He had been feeling down about himself, his career and his direction – a bit of a midlife crisis, if you will. This was spilling out into his relationship too, he was distracted and isolated himself from his family, and mostly from his wife. She thought a fitness routine might help him get his spark back.

His wife was an incredibly wise woman, because *what a great shout*. Not only did exercise help Fred regain his spark – a new-found confidence and new routine – he also had a eureka moment that most likely saved his marriage. Once he was filling up his own cup, he felt much more present and able to fill up his family's cups – and especially his wife's. You know what they say: an empty jug can't pour.

Fred had been running on empty for so long, so it was no wonder he had nothing to give those around him. But fitness changed all of that. His spark for life returned, allowing him to put more energy into the relationship and person he loved most in the world. And an amazing unexpected benefit? His wife started to join him in his gym sessions and on his runs – meaning an extra dimension of their bond together. We simply love to see it.

If you can show up to your fitness regime, you can do the same in your relationships and in your career. You can put your best foot forward, stay present and be the best possible version of yourself. Oh yes, you can!

Fitness encourages a beginner's mindset

We have already touched on this before, so excuse me for repeating myself. When it comes to fitness, everyone has to start somewhere. Even the most successful athlete you know had a time where they had never even tried their sport before, let alone become skilled at it. And this mentality is applicable to everyday life, too. You can't expect to be an expert at anything straight away. No one is born with all the skills and all the answers. Sure, natural talent can come into play, but so much of success is about working hard, trying harder and embracing being a beginner.

This mindset served my client, Jenny*, really well. She had an incredible idea for a business and she dreamed day and night about starting it. But she didn't know the first thing about running a business, so she was afraid to start from scratch and give it a go. And, would you believe it, she also didn't know the first thing about *running* when we first met. A few months later, she was a running pro.

So, what did that teach her? Well, just because she didn't know everything right now about running a business, it didn't mean she never would. She could start from the beginning. She could learn on the go and fail a little along the way – just like she did with running. Suddenly the idea of starting her own business as a little side hustle didn't seem so daunting. She'd been a beginner before, so who said she couldn't be a beginner again? Now, she has a thriving business. 'I genuinely think running gave me the confidence to take the leap,' she told me, and I don't doubt it.

Lessons that last a lifetime

You may have noticed that a few of the points above overlap. Confidence makes it easier to show up as our best selves, and showing up as our best selves can make it easier to do hard things and overcome challenges. It's difficult to separate them (no matter how hard I have tried) because there truly is one big melting pot of benefits to be gained from fitness. Exercise is packed with transferable skills that you can apply to the rest of your life. Maybe you have noticed some other benefits that I haven't mentioned here. What unexpected changes have *you* noticed since starting your fitness journey?

FEAR: RECOVERY IS JUST AS IMPORTANT AS MOVEMENT

You might have thought the final 'fear' section would involve something universally massive and scary, like doing a skydive or jumping off a cliff. As a result, you might be thinking, 'errr, is recovery meant to be scary?'

Well, it might not be for you – and that's great. But I have found that the more you delve into your fitness plan, the more you're busy, busy, busy – setting goals and making strides – the more recovery becomes a fear. Slowing down, taking it easy, healing in between workouts, all of that can get harder and harder to do when you're really in the flow. There's the fear of losing all your progress. You might worry that stopping, even for a little bit, means falling behind and losing steam.

I think it's because of the culture we live in. We're often told that 'doing nothing' is lazy or unproductive. Many of us feel guilty if we just stop and slow down (I have definitely felt this myself). But I want to show you that this is so far from the case. Recovery in between movement is *just as important* as the movement itself. (Read that again, until it properly sinks in.) If you pause your movement and just slow down for a bit, that's definitely not lazy, and it's absolutely not unproductive. That's recovery, darlings!

This is a lesson that I took a while to learn. You already know about my obsession with pushing harder and the spinal injury that led to, so I won't bore you again with the details. We've also discussed how important recovery is for injury prevention and keeping your body safe. But to me, recovery is so much more than that. It's about treating your body with care and respect. It's about giving yourself – your muscles, your mind and your soul – the breathing room you deserve, so you can come back even stronger and enhance your performance.

Non-stop movement leads to burnout, injury and stress. Resting, healing and recovering leads to balance, full-body health and gradual improvement over time. You don't always realise just how important rest is until you're forced to take it. My own experience of extended recovery taught me a hugely important lesson:

sometimes, less is more. I hope you can take this on board *now*, so you don't have to learn the hard way!

I realised that more movement doesn't always equal more benefit. Think of your body a bit like a car. You can't just keep filling up and filling up the tank with petrol, otherwise it would overflow. There's a maximum for a reason, as this is what the car needs to perform at its best. We are the same as cars (sort of). You don't want to fill yourself with movement until you break down. It's all about maintaining steady, healthy levels. That's the aim of the game, my friends.

There are multiple different ways to think about recovery. I like to think it has three sub-categories, which are all extremely important in their own ways: DAILY RECOVERY, WEEKLY RECOVERY and SPECIAL OCCASION RECOVERY.

The first, and most essential, aspect of recovery is the rest you should be having every single day – and that's *sleep*.

The second is the weekly recovery. These are the pockets in your week where you resist the urge to go ham and push yourself to your limits, and instead take time to slow down and reset. Also extremely important.

And finally, you have special occasion recovery. These are recovery techniques you should call upon as and when you need them. Perhaps if you're feeling a little sore, you're training for something big, recovering from injury or you just want to give your body a little extra TLC (because you deserve it, honey).

Now, I'm going to get into each of these recovery types in a little more detail.

DAILY RECOVERY (more commonly known as sleep)

Back when I was an immature little whippersnapper, I believed that sleep was for the weak. '*I'll sleep when I'm dead!*' said ol' Tommy

Trotter of yore, which was truly the incorrect attitude – I can tell you that for free.

Sleeping soundly in your bed each night isn't just a nice-to-have, it's our bodies' way of resting and repairing. As well as being essential for our mental cognition, ability to concentrate and energy levels, it also aids our *physical* recovery, allowing our muscles and bones to recuperate before we put even more pressure on them the next day. Sleep gives our bodies breathing room, a chance to heal from all the stress we've been putting them under.

I have really noticed the difference in how I feel – and how I train – when I don't get my 7–9 hours of sleep (as recommended by the NHS). You know when you've had one too many drinks and the thought of exercising makes you want to hurl? Sleep deprivation can have a similar effect. It makes sense – when you're super tired, everything is going to feel that bit slower, that bit weaker, that bit more sluggish. Although working out can *give you energy* when you're tired, it definitely helps to ensure you're doing the number one thing for your energy levels before you even arrive in the room. And that's getting enough shut-eye.

'But Tom! I have a terrible two-year old/I work shifts/my dog wakes me up at 5am without fail!' I hear you, and this is a common complaint I receive from my clients, too. They're all extremely busy people, with tons of responsibilities that can get in the way of that all-important sleep. It might not always be possible to achieve those 7–9 hours, but all you can do is your best to strive towards that number.

Here are some of my top tips for getting *more* sleep and, importantly, more *good-quality* sleep.

Get into bed earlier. I know this one might seem obvious, but so few of us actually do it. I'm not saying you actually need to go to sleep at 9 p.m. on the dot (although that would be lovely), but if you get yourself totally ready for bed, pyjamas on, teeth brushed, makeup off (if you wear it), then you're getting your body in the zone for sleep. You might watch a TV show (but choose wisely, don't go for something gruesome or intense, as this can be over-stimulating), or read a book (may I recommend this one?), or even listen to a podcast. But just get yourself ready for snoozing, lights dimmed (or off), chilling out. This sends the signal to your brain that sleep is on the horizon, making it easier to come by when you finally lie down.

Stop scrolling. Notice how I didn't include 'scroll mindlessly on TikTok' as a good pre-bedtime activity? That's because scrolling can be overstimulating, keeping your brain awake and therefore preventing it from fully relaxing. I'm obviously not saying you should delete all your social media apps – social media is a big part of my job, after all – but be mindful about how and when you're using it. In the half an hour (or even hour) before bed? Probably not the best idea. Give your poor brain a break! You can catch up on your feed tomorrow!

Prep, prep, prep. Get your meals ready in advance. Get your clothes ready in advance. Get your workout kit ready to go. Whatever you can do during the day to prep you for the next morning is a win, because it means you can have more sleep in the morning. I say this to my clients all the time, and it's often met with resistance. *'But I don't have time to prep!'* they cry. But here's the thing – prepping is short-term effort for long-term gain. And you can easily find ways to make it feel less like a chore. For example, cooking your meal prep or preparing your breakfast at the same time as cooking your dinner. Or planning all your weekly workout sessions before you start your first. Reduce the amount of decisions you need to make in the mornings and you're rewarded with more sleep. Work smarter, not harder!

Watch your caffeine and alcohol intake. As you know, I love a flat white and a G&T as much as the next person, but be mindful about how much you're consuming, and *when* you're consuming it. Coffee is a stimulant that can easily disrupt your sleep if you're drinking it close to bedtime. It also stays in your system for a really long time, so the safest option is to have your last coffee 6–8 hours before bedtime (which is around 12–2 p.m. for most people). Alcohol also might help you fall asleep quicker but it's a sleep-disruptor, reducing the quality of your sleep. The solution on boozy nights? Stop drinking a few hours before sleep, to give your body time to metabolise and break down the alcohol.

Do your thang. We all have our own tried-and-true sleep helpers. Maybe that's spraying lavender on your pillow, or having a cup of herbal tea, doing a little journal exercise to offload any anxieties, or listening to a sleep story or meditation. Whatever you go for, choose something that works for you. What works for one might not work for another person, and that's completely okay. Whatever you do, just make it a priority. Remember sleep ain't for the weak. It's actually for the very strong and very wise.

WEEKLY RECOVERY (Enjoy that blimmin' day off!)

In the past, I've been the kind of guy who would just train, train, train. No days off! No slowing down! My injury forced me to reevaluate that approach. My new approach is to take the damn breaks. Instead of letting my tank overflow, I now try to fill up my tank with 80 per cent of effort – not even to the maximum. This means you'll always have a bit of extra room for a top-up, and you're not going overboard. Think of it a bit like giving your body some wiggle room.

Essentially, this is about slowing down before your body forces you to. If you're feeling a bit sore or tired, listen to that signal your body is sending you. Don't just push through, as you'll end up feeling worse later (either physically or mentally – or both).

This was starting to happen to my client, Seb*. Before starting his programme with me, Seb's issue was recovering a little *too* much (which is to say, he basically didn't exercise at all). But it's funny how, when you get into the rhythm of moving regularly, this becomes your default – and then the reverse happens. It's harder to stop or slow down. Seb started training for a half marathon and was concerned about his progress, so he ran every day for a week. At the end of the week, he felt so burnt out, sore and exhausted that he had to take *two weeks off.* Seb realised that if he just paced himself he wouldn't need to take any chunks of time off – all he needed to do was rest in between sessions. Thankfully he learned his lesson in the nick of time, spacing out his training from that point forward (most running plans recommend around three sessions per week, to give yourself ample recovery time in between).

In my opinion, the average Joe needs about two days per week to focus on recovery, but you might find you need more than that, especially at first. Everyone is different, and so are our recovery times. Experienced athletes may need a little less, but even then, recovery is not to be skipped.

Your recovery days might look different each time. Here are a few ways in which you can recover on a weekly basis:

Just not doing anything. This is especially helpful if your muscles are sore and you've been going ham all week. A complete day off without any movement at all is totally fine. Go on, put your feet up!

Gentle yoga or stretching. Whether it's a hatha or yin class, or just doing some gentle yoga stretches in your living room, this can be a great way to give your muscles some TLC in between workouts.

Swimming or floating. If you have access to a swimming pool in your local gym or leisure centre, it can be great to utilise this regularly for your recovery days. Again, this isn't about whipping out your breaststroke and swimming lengths. Gentle movement in the water, floating and bobbing around is a great way to reset.

Massage guns and bubble baths. We already touched on these in the section on injury (see page 102), but here's a reminder that you can have a spa day from home any time you like. A warm bath (complete with Epsom salts) and a little moment with a massage gun or roller can leave you feeling good as gold.

SPECIAL OCCASION RECOVERY (take it as you need it)

There are some recovery options that are a little more expensive – either because they're highly specialised and a bit more medical, or they're just a bit boujie and luxurious. You really don't have to pay for these options unless you need them, or just want a treat. Still, there's so much out there that you can try.

Physio. Super important if you have an injury or a niggle. Depending on what your issue is, you may be able to get this on the NHS. Otherwise, there are plenty of sports physios who can provide services as one-offs.

Massage. If the massage gun is just not hitting the spot, or you need a more specialised sports massage from an experienced professional, it could be worth booking one. Just make sure you look for a reputable place.

Flotation tanks. This is a really cool form of recovery – you simply float in a tank that's filled with salts so you become completely weightless. Not only are these incredibly calming for the mind, they're also relaxing for the muscles, especially taking pressure off the back and neck.

Cryotherapy/Ice baths. Mega-cold temperatures are a little controversial when it comes to recovery, but so many athletes swear by this approach. I, for one, love the invigorating feeling you get from dunking into an ice bath, and I do think my muscles feel great afterwards. Each to their own – and make sure you do it safely!

Sauna. The same goes with high heats as a form of recovery – the science isn't always super clear, but if it feels good to you to sweat profusely, then go for it. Again, make sure you do it safely – never spend longer than 15 minutes in a sauna, and stay hydrated.

Fill up your cup

Repeat after me: I am allowed to recover and recovery is not a failure. Whether you feel sick as a dog, your period is due or you're healing from an injury – you should always feel comfortable taking breaks, slowing down and giving your body the love and appreciation it deserves. Filling up your cup doesn't mean jam-packing it with movement, goals and targets. It also means filling it with rest, love and a sense of ease. When you get the balance right between movement and rest, you know you're onto a winner.

FITNESS: YOUR 14-DAY FITNESS CHALLENGE

Wowee, what a journey. If you've made it to this fitness section you've already covered a lot of ground. You know how to incorporate movement into your everyday life, build strength with your body weight, machines and dumbbells, run and cycle, embrace high-intensity bursts and low-intensity exercise (like Pilates and yoga) too. You're *basically* a fitness expert – which means you're ready to participate in my (drum roll please) 14-DAY FITNESS CHALLENGE!

Don't be alarmed, this challenge is not about pushing you to your absolute limits every single day. That would contradict our last section on recovery, wouldn't it? This is simply a format that covers everything you've learned so far, allowing you to see your progression and show yourself what is possible. If you get through this challenge in one piece, and you love it, then feel free to repeat it as much as you want, adapting it to suit your individual preferences. This is *your* journey – and you're more than capable of taking the wheel.

You can start this challenge at any time – on a Monday or a Wednesday or in the middle of the night. Most of the workouts require no specialist kit, except gym clothes and an exercise mat. However, a couple of them will recommend dumbbells (but if you don't have any, you can use tins of baked beans or something similar), and I've also suggested resistance bands for one of them, but this is optional. If you've been doing all the fitness sections in this book, you'll already recognise most of these exercises, so nothing should feel *too far* outside of your comfort zone. I have also included progressions, and easier versions, of moves wherever possible. Remember to listen to your body, do what you can, and *have fun*.

Let's go!!

NOTE: I haven't included warm-up and cool-downs in these exercises. For my easy-peasy, use anytime warm-ups and cool-downs, head to page 105.

DAY 1: EASY-PEASY 30-MINUTE RUN

This is exactly what it says on the tin – 30 minutes of chilled running. I've done this by time and not by distance so that it's more about time on feet, getting your heart rate up and seeing what you can do rather than pushing yourself to cover a certain amount of ground. Whether you run 1k or 8k in this time, all are totally fine. But I'd recommend purposely going a bit slower on this run as you'll need the warm-up for the rest of the week. Jog at a conversational pace, focusing on your posture and breath.

DAY 2: 20-MINUTE UPPER BODY STRENGTH

This simple upper body strength exercise uses only four of my favourite moves – each one using dumbbells (if you can). These moves cover all the most important muscles in your upper body (the ones that make you look jacked) including your upper back, shoulders, traps, biceps and triceps. You'll complete 10–12 reps of each move for one set, take 30–45 seconds rest in between sets, then repeat the set again twice more.

Make sure you choose weights that will allow you to complete all the reps – but the last two should feel difficult! If you can barely do the first few, they're too heavy. If you're getting to the end too easily, they're too light.

Shoulder press (3 sets of 10). Stand or sit upright with a dumbbell in each hand, at shoulder height, with your palms facing forward.

Engage your core as you press the weights upwards until your arms are fully extended overhead. Then slowly lower back down to shoulder height. (See page 53.)

Bent-over rows (3 sets of 12). From standing, hold a dumbbell in each hand, with your palms facing your body. Hinge at your hips with a slight bend in your knees, keeping your back flat (no arching) and your chest up. Let your arms hang straight down towards the ground, then lift the dumbbells up towards your ribcage, squeezing your shoulder blades together. Slowly lower back down and repeat.

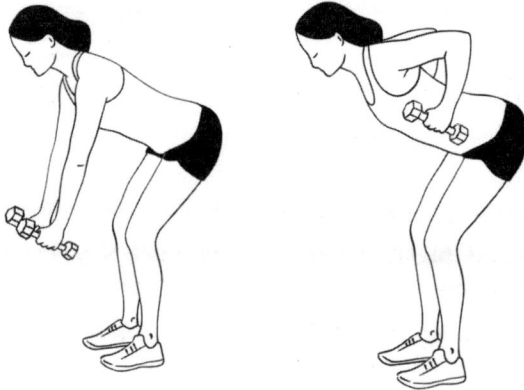

Bicep curls (3 sets of 10). Start with the dumbbells at your sides, with your palms facing forwards. Keeping your elbows close to your body, curl your dumbbells up to shoulder height, activating your biceps. Slowly lower back down with control. (See page 52.)

Tricep kickbacks (3 sets of 10). Start in a similar way to the bent-over row: holding a dumbbell in each hand and hingeing forward at the hips. Bend your elbows to 90 degrees so that your upper arms are close to your torso. While keeping your upper arms still, straighten your arms back behind you to 'kick back' the weights. Squeeze at the top, then return slowly. (See page 53.)

DAY 3: 20-MINUTE LOWER BODY STRENGTH

Why complicate things if we don't need to? This lower body strength workout follows the same format as the upper body workout you completed yesterday – just four moves and three sets of each move, with 45 seconds of rest in between each set. These moves will target all the main parts of your lower body – including glutes, hamstrings, quads, calves and hip flexors.

You can do these moves using just your body weight, but I will show you how you can add in dumbbells for progression. Remember, you might be able to go a bit heavier with these dumbbells than you did with your upper body exercises.

Squats (3 sets of 12). You can either hold out your hands in front of you or hold a single dumbbell with both hands, *or* hold two dumbbells by your sides. Stand with your feet shoulder-width apart, toes turned out slightly. Lower down by bending at the hips and knees and engaging your core, being sure to keep your chest up and your knees tracking over your toes. Lower down until your thighs are as close to parallel with the ground as possible, then push through your heels with control to stand back up. Avoid leaning forward as much as possible, to maintain proper form! (See page 25.)

Alternating lunges (3 sets of 10). You can do this without weights, or hold dumbbells in each hand down by your sides. If not using weights, you may want to place your hands on your hips for balance. From standing, step one foot forward and bend both knees to around 90 degrees. Keep your front knee over your ankle and your back knee hovering above the ground. Push back to standing through that standing leg, then switch sides. Keep alternating – doing 5 on each side for a single set. (See page 24.)

Glute bridges (3 sets of 15). Lie on your back with your knees bent, feet flat and legs hip-width apart. If you're using a dumbbell for this, hold a dumbbell on your hips (resting across your pelvis). If not, have your arms by your sides. Press down on your heels to lift your hips until your body forms a straight line from your shoulders to your knees. Squeeze those glutes at the top, then lower down slowly. (See page 49.)

Calf raises (3 sets of 12). Stand with your feet hip-width apart – ideally near a chair or wall for balance. If you're opting for dumbbells, hold one in each hand by your sides. Press through the balls of your feet to lift your heels off the ground. Pause at the top, then slowly lower down. As the name suggests, you should really feel this in your calves! (See page 23.)

DAY 4: 10-MINUTE YOGA STRETCH

After all that strength-building, it's time to cool it down with some gentle stretches that just feel so. Damn. *Good.* Move slowly through each of these poses, holding each for roughly 2 minutes. You can fit this in whenever you like, but it might feel especially nice to do it before bedtime, to prep your body and mind for sleep.

Move slowly through these yoga poses, holding each one for 2 minutes, breathing deeply throughout.

Child's pose. Starting on your hands and knees (tabletop position), bring your big toes to touch and your knees wide. Sit your bum back towards your heels. Stretch your arms out in front of you, resting your forehead on the ground. Breathe deeply, and sway side to side if that feels good. Place a cushion or block under your head if that feels more comfortable. (See page 169.)

Cat cow. Starting in tabletop, inhale as you arch your back, lift your bum, drop your belly and look up (for cow pose). Then exhale as you round your spine, tucking in your pelvis, drawing your belly in and looking down (for cat pose). Keep going, and don't be afraid to veer off the tracks, wiggling and moving however feels good to you. Pause in any places that feel like a good stretch for you. (See page 82.)

Downward dog. Starting in tabletop (or a high plank if you want a bit more spice), tuck in your toes, lift your knees off the ground, sending your hips up and back, forming a sort-of triangle. Straighten your legs and back as much as you can, but it's okay to have a slight bend in the knees and for your heels to be lifted. Stretch out in a way that feels good – then take your dog for a walk by slowly lowering the heels. You may also want to look under each armpit for more of a twist. (See page 83.)

Seated forward fold. This will feel amazing after working those hamstrings and calves yesterday! Sit down with your legs extended in front of you and feet flexed. Straighten your legs if you can, but it's also okay to keep your legs bent if you have tight hamstrings and it feels more comfortable. Inhale, sit up tall, then exhale while hingeing from your hips and reaching towards your feet. Don't round your upper back, keep your spine long. Only reach as far as is comfy for you – it's totally fine if your arms only reach your thighs (you will build more flexibility over time and this will get easier!).

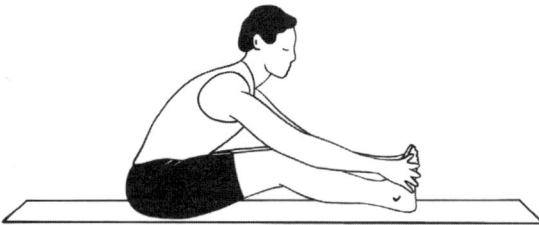

Supine twist. This twisty stretch will feel great in your back. Lie on your back with your legs extended, then hug one knee into your chest before crossing it over your body, letting the leg rest on the floor on the opposite side. Extend the other arm to the side and gaze in that direction. Relax, breathing deeply, then switch sides when you're about halfway through. (See page 109.)

DAY 5: 10-MINUTE AB BLAST

Fancy a six-pack in 10 minutes?! (Well, I can't promise a six-pack after the first time you do this . . . but if you do it repeatedly, you'll be well on your way!) These exercises will strengthen your ab muscles for a sculpted look, but, most importantly, they will also strengthen your core, which will then support all other forms of movement.

Simply do three rounds of each of the following, with 30 seconds of rest in between.

30-second plank (repeat 3 times). You can choose to do this as a forearm plank (with elbows down, resting on your forearms), or a high plank (hands on the floor). If doing a forearm plank, your elbows should be in line with your shoulders; for a high plank, your hands should be in line. From your chosen arm position, extend your legs back, forming a straight line from your head to your heels. Engage your core, squeeze those glutes and keep your neck neutral (no unnecessary tensing!). Hold for 30 seconds, breathing steadily (this will make it feel easier – trust me). If you want to take it easier, keep your knees on the floor for a supported plank. (See page 25.)

15 bicycle crunches (repeat 3 times). Lie on your back with your knees bent, your head, neck and shoulders slightly off the ground. Put your hands by your head, or hands around your neck for added support. Bring your right elbow towards your left knee as you extend the right leg. Then switch sides, bringing your left elbow towards your right knee while extending the left leg. Keep going in a pedalling motion until you've done 15 on each side. The quicker you go, the harder it will be – just be sure that speed doesn't mean losing your form. (See page 167.)

10 Russian twists (repeat 3 times). Sit on the floor with your knees bent and feet either flat or lifted slightly off the ground (lifted will be harder!). Lean back slightly, keeping your spine straight and chest lifted. Hold your hands together (or a dumbbell) and rotate your torso so that you tap the floor beside your hip. Twist to the other side. Keep going until you've done 10 on each side (20 total). If your back is hurting, sit more upright. (See page 142.)

15 leg raises (repeat 3 times). Lie flat on your back with legs straight and arms at your sides. Keep your legs together and straight, lifting them towards the ceiling as vertical and high as you possibly can. Slowly lower your legs back down without letting your lower back arch or lift off the floor. Repeat another 15 times to complete the set. (See page 84.)

DAY 6: CHOOSE-YOUR-OWN 60-MINUTE CARDIO

If you're not a fan of running, this is the cardio day for you. Choose your own adventure – whether that's getting out on your bike or opting for a cardio gym machine (see the options on page 116).

Try to keep this as steady-state as possible – meaning you're maintaining a fairly consistent pace. Choose a pace that you can consistently keep for 60 full minutes. But, of course, listen to your body; if you need to slow down or walk for some of it, then absolutely do that. Take breaks as and when you need.

The challenge is to get your heart rate up, work up a sweat and push through the pain (and sometimes the boredom) of a long session. You've got this! I believe in you!

DAY 7: RECOVERY DAY

This is another choose-your-own adventure day! Either take the day off or do some very gentle movement (like swimming) if it's accessible and you fancy it. But it's totally okay to just sleep an extra hour too. No guilt allowed.

DAY 8: 20-MINUTE FULL-BODY STRENGTH

You've done upper body, lower body and abs, so now it's time to target your whole body in one go. These four moves work multiple different muscles across your body, including your legs, arms, back and core. You'll be super-strong and ready to support your body through some cardio tomorrow!

This time, complete just 2 rounds of each exercise, taking a 60-minute rest in between each round. These exercises use a lot of energy, so utilise that extra break time to calm your body and stay hydrated. This workout is best completed with dumbbells, but you don't need to use them if you don't have any.

10 walk-outs (repeat twice). Stand tall, with your feet hip-width apart. Hinge at your hips and walk your hands forward into a high plank. For the advanced version, you can add in a push-up here, either with your knees down or up on your toes. Lower your chest slowly to the floor. Or you can simply skip this part and walk your hands back to your feet to stand. Then repeat. (See page 46.)

10 squats-to-press (repeat twice). Holding a dumbbell in each hand at shoulder height, lower down into a squat (sitting back into a chair with your knees tracking over your toes and your chest up). As you rise up, press the weights up overhead, straightening your arms. Then lower your weights back down to your shoulders as you move into the next squat. You can also do this without dumbbells, simply lifting your arms up explosively.

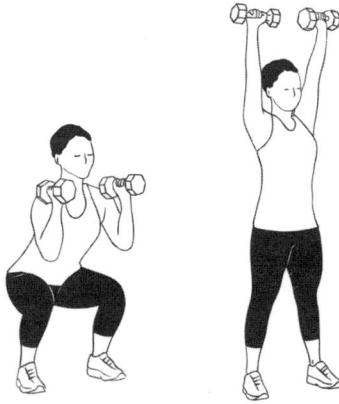

20 standing woodchoppers (repeat twice). This is a great rotational and full-body move that gets you working your obliques (the sides of your core – which we can easily ignore). Stand with your feet shoulder-width apart, holding one dumbbell in both hands. Begin with the weight high above one shoulder – then, in one controlled movement, twist your torso and bring the weight diagonally across your body to the outside of your opposite hip. Return to your starting position. Do 10 reps on one side before switching to the other side.

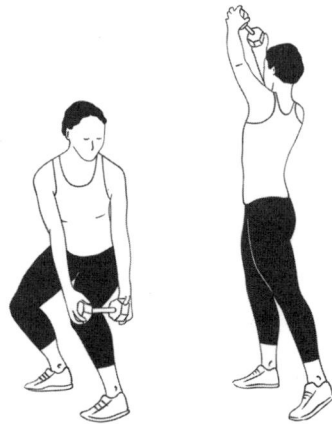

199

10 deadlifts (repeat twice). Hold two dumbbells in front of your thighs. With a slight bend in your knees, hinge at your hips to lower the weights down in front of your legs. Keep your back flat and your shoulders pulled back, then engage your glutes to return to standing. Remember: the movement comes from your hips – you should feel this in your glutes, hamstrings and lower back.

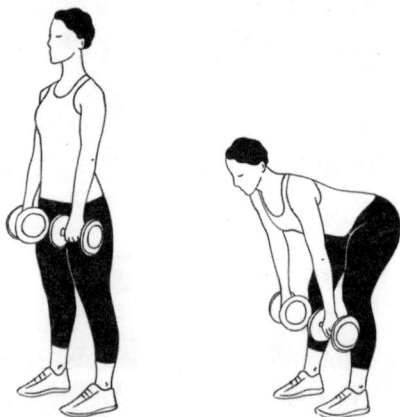

DAY 9: HIIT RUNNING SPRINTS (FOR 45 MINUTES)

You've done some easy and steady-state cardio, now it's time to put a rocket up your butt and increase the intensity. This work-out will see you do some fast sprints, but don't worry, you're not expected to maintain that speed for too long, as you'll have walk-ing intervals. Knowing you have a walking break coming up will (hopefully) allow you to push yourself to your edge during the sprint. Expect to finish this workout feeling sweaty and pumped full of endorphins.

First, plan your route – it could be a good shout to pick a park or promenade where you can do loops, so you don't need to think about where you're going next. Or you can use a treadmill if you'd prefer.

Warm up with a 10-minute steady-state walk or jog. If you're jogging, make sure you could still hold a conversation while you move.

Your intervals are going to look like this: 30 seconds of running at full pelt – as fast as you possibly can – followed by a 90-second walk in between. You may want to jog slightly on either side of the walk to ease yourself in and out of those fast 30 seconds. Repeat this 10 times.

Once you're done, finish off with a 10-minute easy walk, and complete a few stretches (see my cool-down on page 107).

DAY 10: 10-MINUTE BOOTY BURN

This is gonna be a toughie after two days of going ham. But this workout is only 10 minutes, and I believe you have it in you to get it done. You'll feel so proud of yourself afterwards.

This quickie is all about working your glutes. For these moves, you can use only your body weight or a resistance band. I'll show you how they'll work with each. This workout includes just 3 different moves – you're going to repeat 3 rounds, with 30 seconds of rest in between each round.

20 donkey kicks (repeat 3 times). Start from a tabletop position: hands under your shoulders, knees under hips and your back flat. If you're doing the more advanced version, place a looped resistance band around your thighs. Shift your weight slightly to one side, then lift the other leg off the ground, keeping it bent at 90 degrees. Press your foot up and back towards the ceiling, lifting your thigh until it's in line with your upper body. Squeeze your glute at the top, trying not to arch your back. Slowly return to the start but keep your knee hovering slightly off the ground. Repeat 10 times before switching to the other side.

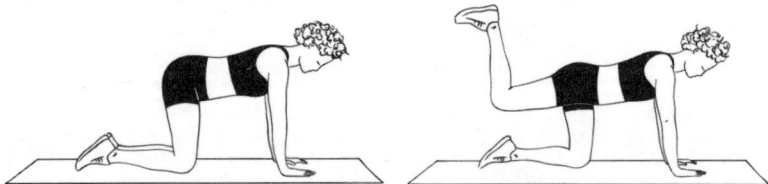

20 fire hydrants (repeat 3 times). Staying on all fours, you can do this move with body weight alone, or move your resistance band down to just above your knees. Keeping your knee bent at 90 degrees, lift it out to the side – similar to the donkey kicks, except this time you're using the side of your glutes. Only lift as far as you can go while still keeping your hips square. Pause briefly at the top, then lower down gently with control – again, not resting the knee fully on the ground. Repeat 10 times before switching to the other side.

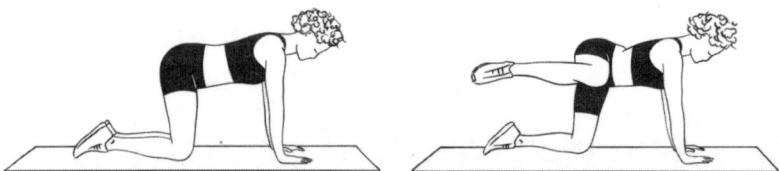

20 Bulgarian split squats (repeat 3 times). For this move, you'll need a low bench, step or a sturdy chair. You can also hold dumbbells in each hand if you like, or go without. Stand a few feet in front of your bench, step or chair, and place your back foot on the bench – with the top of the foot flat, or toes tucked under. Then hop your front foot forward so you're in a stable lunge position. Lean forward slightly, as this will keep the focus in your glutes.

Lower down until your front thigh is parallel to the ground, with your knee stacked over your ankle. Drive through the front heel to stand back up. Complete 10 on one side before switching over.

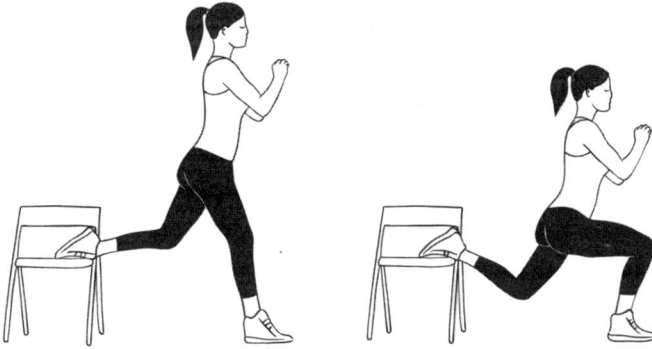

DAY 11: CHILLED 'N' VIBEY 60-MINUTE WALK

Think of this as a bonus recovery day – all you're going to do is get outside in nature and enjoy an easy-breezy walk. Slowly moving will help any sore muscles you're feeling from yesterday's booty burn. Either plug into some music or your favourite podcast, or drag a friend out to meet you so you can walk and yap.

DAY 12: 15-MINUTE CORE-OF-STEEL PILATES

This Pilates workout will give you a full-body burn, but with a specific focus on building your core strength while also marrying the breath with movement. It's not about the number of reps you do – this is all about quality over quantity. Each round will last 40 seconds, and you'll do three rounds of each move, switching sides after 20 seconds each time, and with 20 seconds of rest in between each round.

203

Dead bug (for 40 seconds, repeat 3 times). Lie on your back, with knees in tabletop position and your arms extended straight up. Lower one arm and the opposite leg at the same time, keeping your back firmly pressed into the mat. Return to your starting position, then switch sides. Move slowly, with control, exhaling each time you extend and inhaling each time you return. (See page 51.)

Single leg stretch (for 40 seconds, repeat 3 times). Lying on your back, lift up your head and pull your knees into your chest. Extend one leg out while lightly holding the opposite shin. Switch legs so that you flow between the moves seamlessly. If you're feeling it in your neck, lower your head back down to the ground.

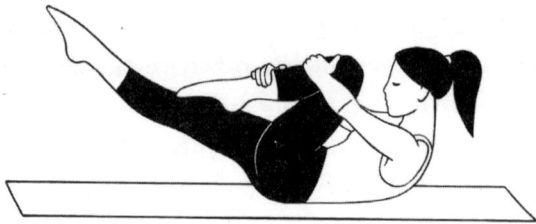

Side plank and reach (for 40 seconds, repeat 3 times). Now let's work those obliques! Start in a side plank on your right side – get into this by lying on your right side, legs extended and stacked on top of each other. With your elbow directly under your shoulder and forearm parallel to the top of your mat, engage your core and lift your hips off the mat so your body is in a straight line from head to heels. Keep your top shoulder stacked over the bottom (try not to roll forward or back). If this feels too difficult, you can place your top foot on the ground for support. From this position, extend your top arm to the sky, then thread it under your torso before returning.

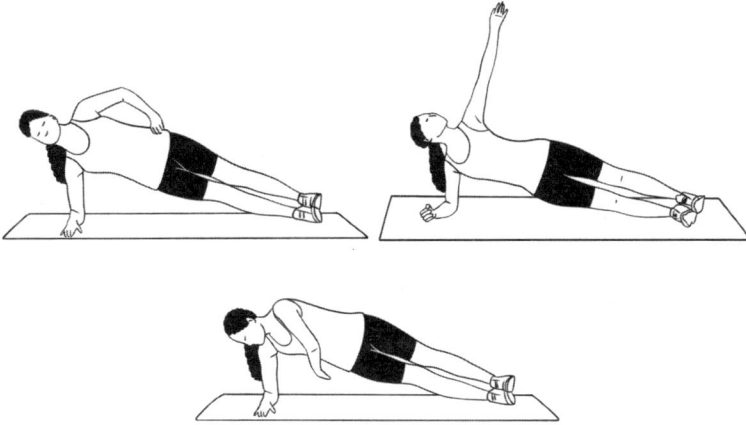

Side-lying leg lifts (for 40 seconds, repeat 3 times). Lie on one side with your legs straight and stacked. Your head can be raised, with your hand holding it up, or placed down on the mat. Lift up your top leg slowly, then lower it back down with control. You might want to keep your top hand on your hip to maintain alignment and avoid rocking back. Bonus: Add in 10 small pulses at the top for the final few seconds of each side.

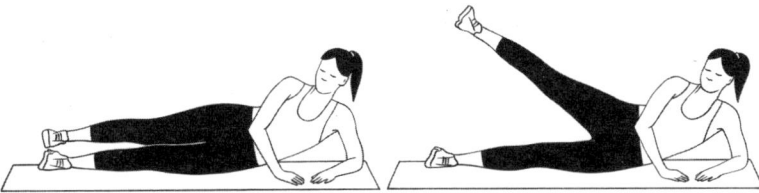

DAY 13: 30-MINUTE SWEAT-FEST

Let's finish off this challenge on a high, shall we? And when I say high, I'm talking high intensity. Think speed, power and endurance. Oh yeah, baby!

In this workout, you're going to complete each set of a move and then head straight into the next one – no resting in between. But don't worry, you get 1 minute's rest between each round, and you'll complete three circuits in total. Stay hydrated and keep your head in the game.

10 jump squats. Stand with your feet shoulder-width apart, then lower into a squat – hips back, knees tracking over toes, chest up. From the bottom of the squat, push upwards into an explosive squat, swinging your arms to create momentum. Land as softly as possible (to protect those knees), then immediately move into the next squat. (See page 164.)

10 push-ups. Either do these on your knees or go full-pelt with your legs extended and toes tucked under. Lower your chest to the floor by bending your elbows at a 45-degree angle, then push back up. (See page 166.)

10 dumbbell (or kettlebell) swings. Stand with your feet shoulder-width apart, holding a dumbbell (or kettlebell) with both hands. Hinge at the hips to swing the dumbbell back between your legs. Then thrust your hips forward with power to swing the dumbbell up to shoulder height before letting it swing back naturally. Make sure this movement is coming from your hips, not your knees or your arms!

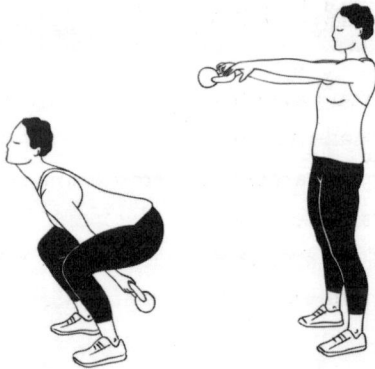

20 mountain climbers (10 on each side). Starting in a high-plank position (hands under shoulders, body in a straight line from head to heels), drive your right knee to your chest then switch legs. Alternate your legs quickly as if you're running in place. Try to keep your hips low and your core tight to avoid bouncing around and losing stability. You can also slow them down for more control. (See page 49.)

20-second spring or high knees. If you're in a gym, you can use a treadmill, or if you're at home, simply run in place. Sprint for 20 seconds at the maximum effort you can muster, or jog in place, driving your knees up towards your chest as high as you can. Once you're finished, take a 1-minute rest, before repeating the whole circuit again. And then again. (Trust me, you can do it.)

DAY 14: RECOVERY DAY

YOU MADE IT! Go wild with your recovery today. Book a massage. Go to a sauna. Have an extended nap. Let your mind and body rest completely – whatever that means to you. You've earned it.

FUN: LIVE IT AND BREATHE IT, EVERY DAY

So, here we are. You have officially made it through every level of my plan. You've made it through the tricky beginning stages when everything feels unbearably hard. You've made it through all the mindset blockers, the excuses and the fears. You've learned about parts of yourself that you never knew existed. You found a rhythm and you discovered resilience. This, my friend, is where the fun begins.

You don't have a fun activity for this chapter because now you're going to start living and breathing this healthy lifestyle that you've begun to build. Living healthily, committed to exercise and becoming the best version of yourself can be hard, but it's also blimmin' fun. There's truly nothing more fun than riding off on that magical unicorn, taking on your days with ambition, motivation and a lust for life. Now, it's not a part of yourself that you're trying to grow. It's *who you are*. You are a unicorn-rider. You don't need to try to rise and shine every day, you simply do it, without thinking.

If you still don't feel like you're quite there yet, that's okay. You can return to any chapter in this book and work through the levels again and again if you need to. As much as I love a good race, *life* is not a race, and you are more than welcome to go as quickly or as slowly as you like. But I *know* that if you stick with me, and you commit to yourself, then you will get to this place eventually. Where you're not forcing, you're not struggling, you're not battling. That doesn't mean it'll never be challenging, only that the idea of challenge becomes second nature. Something to run towards, not run away from. Something that excites you and makes you feel amazing. Eventually, I hope that fitness will remind you just how good it feels to be alive.

Before I leave you to spread your wings and gallop away, I want you to remember these very important points . . .

You are strong.
You are capable.
You are resilient.
You are impressive.
You are inspirational.
. . . and I'm so damn proud of you.

Lots of love,
Tommy x

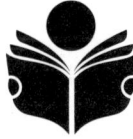

RAISING READERS
Books Build Bright Futures

Dear Reader,

We'd love your attention for one more page to tell you about the crisis in children's reading, and what we can all do.

Studies have shown that reading for fun is the **single biggest predictor of a child's future life chances** – more than family circumstance, parents' educational background or income. It improves academic results, mental health, wealth, communication skills, ambition and happiness.[1]

The number of children reading for fun is in rapid decline. Young people have a lot of competition for their time. In 2024, 1 in 10 children and young people in the UK aged 5 to 18 did not own a single book at home.[2]

Hachette works extensively with schools, libraries and literacy charities, but here are some ways we can all raise more readers:

- Reading to children for just 10 minutes a day makes a difference
- Don't give up if children aren't regular readers – there will be books for them!
- Visit bookshops and libraries to get recommendations
- Encourage them to listen to audiobooks
- Support school libraries
- Give books as gifts

There's a lot more information about how to encourage children to read on our website: **www.RaisingReaders.co.uk**

Thank you for reading.

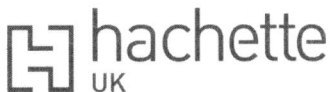

hachette
UK

---

[1] OECD, '21st-Century Readers: Developing Literacy Skills in a Digital World', 2021, https://www.oecd.org/en/publications/21st-century-readers_a83d84cb-en.html

[2] National Literacy Trust, 'Book Ownership in 2024', November 2024, https://literacytrust.org.uk/research-services/research-reports/book-ownership-in-2024

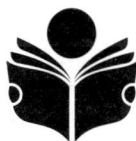

RAISING READERS
Books Build Bright Futures

Dear Reader,

We'd love your attention for one more page to tell you about the crisis in children's reading, and what we can all do.

Studies have shown that reading for fun is the **single biggest predictor of a child's future life chances** – more than family circumstance, parents' educational background or income. It improves academic results, mental health, wealth, communication skills, ambition and happiness.[1]

The number of children reading for fun is in rapid decline. Young people have a lot of competition for their time. In 2024, 1 in 10 children and young people in the UK aged 5 to 18 did not own a single book at home.[2]

Hachette works extensively with schools, libraries and literacy charities, but here are some ways we can all raise more readers:

- Reading to children for just 10 minutes a day makes a difference
- Don't give up if children aren't regular readers – there will be books for them!
- Visit bookshops and libraries to get recommendations
- Encourage them to listen to audiobooks
- Support school libraries
- Give books as gifts

There's a lot more information about how to encourage children to read on our website: **www.RaisingReaders.co.uk**

Thank you for reading.

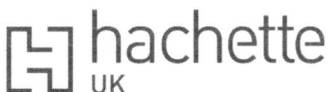

hachette
UK

---

[1] OECD, '21st-Century Readers: Developing Literacy Skills in a Digital World', 2021, https://www.oecd.org/en/publications/21st-century-readers_a83d84cb-en.html

[2] National Literacy Trust, 'Book Ownership in 2024', November 2024, https://literacytrust.org.uk/research-services/research-reports/book-ownership-in-2024